LOST
IN
LYME

LOST IN LYME

The Therapeutic Use
of Medicinal Plants
in Supporting People
with Lyme Disease

Julia Behrens

with
Daphne Lambert

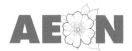

The intent of this book is solely informational and educational. The information and suggestions in this book are not intended to replace the advice or treatments given by health professionals. The author and publisher have made every effort to present accurate information. However, they shall be neither responsible nor liable for any problem that may arise from information in this book.

First published in 2023 by
Aeon Books Ltd

British Library Cataloguing in Publication Data

A C.I.P. for this book is available from the British Library

ISBN: 978–1–80152–012–6

Printed in Great Britain

www.aeonbooks.co.uk

CONTENTS

LIST OF PLANT PROFILES

Julia Behrens is a qualified practitioner in herbal medicine with a degree from the College of Phytotherapy, graduating with honours in 2000. She trained with Hein Zeyelastra. She is a member of the College of Practitioners of Phytotherapy (mCPP) and has diplomas in nutrition and therapeutic massage. Julia has taught at the School of Herbal Medicine, lectured at East London and Westminster universities, consulted for the WWF, and worked at Neal's Yard Remedies. She runs a range of courses in herbal medicine for schools and community groups, including at Phoenix Community Centre, Plumpton College, and the Heartwood Education Foundation. She has published articles about the conservation of medicinal plants in the *European Journal of Herbal Medicine* and for WWF and Plantlife, and is a co-author of *Healing Herbs* (Dorling Kindersley, 2020).

She participates in the Future Health Project, a Brighton-based organisation of GPs, practitioners, community workers, and developers. The project is part of the humanities in future health network at the University of Sussex, bringing together Sussex academics and local health and arts partners to explore ideas for future collaborations in the delivery of health care in the twenty-first century.

She works in clinics in Brighton, Hove, Bristol, and Eastbourne and alongside doctors at the Integrative Herstmonceux Health Centre in Hailsham, where she designed a herb garden for the patients there to use.

Together with Daphne Lambert, she runs a series of workshops for the Greencuisine Trust, including well-women retreats and workshops, raising awareness of plants and food that can help those with Lyme disease.

Julia applies sustainable and holistic principles in both her medicinal practice and treatment of clients. She makes many of the herbal preparations she uses herself, mindful at all times of how the plants were grown and harvested.

She was invited to join and help set up a Lyme clinic at the Herstmonceux Integrative Health Centre, which was established in 2015 with a focus on providing a holistic approach to treating patients with

Lyme disease. She was part of a team with Dr John Simmons and Tanya Borowski, a functional medicine practitioner. The use of bespoke herbal protocols, regular patient discussions, and a collaborative approach to care resulted in the clinic attracting clients from all over the world, with some clients even funding treatment programmes for less fortunate patients. Having all practitioners under one roof allowed for seamless collaboration and a unified approach to patient care. This resulted in a wellness system that ensured each patient received the best possible treatment. Despite its success, the Lyme clinic disbanded in 2017 due to the pressures of working within an NHS setting and the desire of some team members to pursue further research and other interests.

ACKNOWLEDGEMENTS

I owe an enormous debt of gratitude to those many, many people who have supported me in countless ways. My special thanks go to my clients, and sponsors who have trusted me and the herbs and contributed their experience to this book, who have found healing and direction, motivating me to share and continue my work, and whose unheard voices I hope can be heard though these pages.

I am also truly grateful to Tim Hanley, graphic designer, Sophie Gouk Illustrations, and Eric and Klara King for editing who were willing to assist with innovative visual reminders and ideas that enabled me to communicate a complex subject in such a beautiful and comprehensible style.

Special thanks go to Jess Owen, Diana Gobel, Tim Hanley, Ella Lebeau, Kate Jackman, Suzannah Behrens, Peter Scott, Gillian Crowther, Armin Schwarzbach, Mary Wagner, Sarah Anderson, Dr John Simmons, Bea Simmons, Martin Powell, Chris Etheridge, Alison Behrens, Elena Behrens, Mark Bolwell, Jonathan Newman, Oliver Rathbone, and Melinda McDougall.

Above all, extra special thanks go to Matthew, Cass, and Asha, my beloved family who have walked and laughed alongside me. I am deeply indebted to them for giving me space, understanding, and the time to write.

I would especially like to thank Daphne Lambert, for her many years of friendship and for her contributions to writing chapters 8 and 9, and the late Stephen Buhner, both of whose knowledge and understanding of plants truly inspired me and without whose work I may never have found the tools that developed my calling to support the Lyme community, sharing practical solutions to treating Lyme disease.

I would like to thank the following for photographs and illustrations: Sharon Chen (p. 213); Hugo Fox (p. 3); Lynda Kelly (p. 172); Daphne Lambert (pp. 194, 207, 208, 210, 213, 217); Martin Pettit (p. 232); Martin Powell (pp. 54–55); Igor Tudoran (p. 105); Sarah Weal (p. 60); Leo Zoltan (p. 202).

Disclaimer

The information in this book is intended for general information only. It is not intended to amount to advice on which you should rely and is not a substitute for diagnosis by a qualified and experienced health professional.

Any potentially serious health conditions should be evaluated by a qualified health professional. Most herbs and supplements have not been thoroughly tested for their interactions with other foods, herbs, or medications.

I have written this book on the therapeutic use of herbs in the treatment and support of people with Lyme disease to share my knowledge and experience in using herbs alongside conventional treatments.

I also want to educate others on the potential benefits and risks of using herbs in managing Lyme disease and to provide a resource for those seeking alternative or complementary treatments for the condition.

The book can be used as a resource in several ways:

- *Chapter by chapter:* You can read the book cover to cover to gain a comprehensive understanding of the topic.
- *Dip-in approach:* You can use the book as a reference by dipping in and out of different chapters or sections based on your requirements.
- *Plant-specific information:* You can use the book to look up information on individual plants and their use in treating Lyme disease.
- *Client stories:* The book includes client stories, highlighted in green. You can use these as examples to see how others have used herbs or experienced their Lyme disease journey and what results they have achieved.
- *Self-help strategies* for managing Lyme disease, including information on food and nutrition, recipes, essential oils, and pain management.
- *Future developments* in the treatment of Lyme disease, including growing your own medicine.

Once you have gained an understanding of the basics of Lyme disease and the various treatment options available, you may want to consider reaching out to a practitioner for personalized guidance and support. The final chapter, on practitioners, can provide you with information on where to start and what to expect when working with a practitioner.

Remember, taking care of your physical and mental health is an ongoing process, and it is important to work closely with your healthcare provider to develop a comprehensive personalised treatment plan that is right for you.

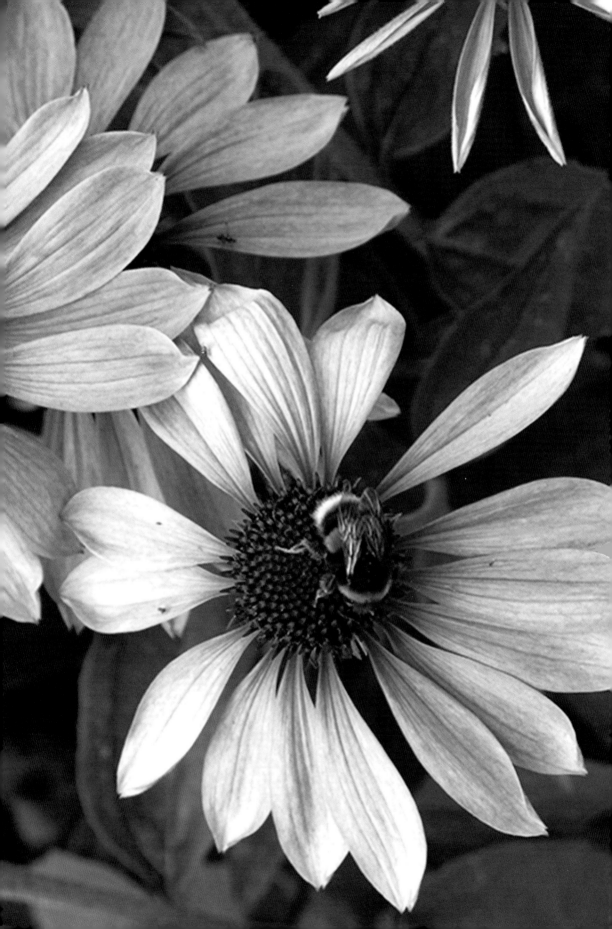

Introduction

It has been my privilege for over 20 years to work with doctors and hundreds of clients who have found that an effective way to treat Lyme disease is herbal medicine. The infection can be quite overwhelming, so this book sets out to offer readers, at a time when they may feel quite lost, a comprehensive overview of the disease and its treatment.

Herbalism, which is both an ancient art and a modern science, is the most widely practised medicine worldwide – the primary form of health care for 80% of the planet, according to the WHO. In the past, it was through trial and error that our ancestors discovered the healing power of plants. Nowadays, a more scientific approach is taken in understanding the medicinal properties of herbs.

Herbal practitioners use diagnostic skills similar to those in orthodox medicine but with preparations made from the whole plant to treat their patients, whereas orthodox practitioners use isolated compounds from plants, or synthetic drugs. A herbal practitioner treats the whole person rather than just the symptoms, based on the philosophy that the suppression of symptoms alone does not lead to complete health, because the underlying problem is not addressed. Herbal medicine can be used both as preventative medicine and as a treatment to improve general health and vitality. It is suitable for people of all ages, from babies to the elderly.

Herbal medicine can be used in a wide range of ways: to help reduce inflammation, manage co-infections, regulate hormones, detoxify, and replace nutrients depleted in the body. Herbal medicine can also help protect the body by enhancing the immune system, reducing the side effects of medications, alleviating symptoms resulting from ill health, and helping to relieve stress.

When, as a child, I had the first signs of a cold or couldn't sleep, my mother would get out a large wooden box, inside which was her domestic apothecary, with herbs and tinctures she used to make teas. She would make an aromatic foaming hot bath with bubbles, sent with love from her home country, Germany. I would drink the herbal tea she made and lie down in the steamy bath. When I could no longer tolerate the heat, I would get out of the bath, and my mother would wrap me in towels and blankets, joking that I was like an embalmed Egyptian mummy. I thought I would melt beneath the covers, but knew I would feel better; eventually I fell asleep, and, within that cocoon, the increase in temperature helped my immune system to respond to the infection.

As long as I can remember I have had plants in my life. I often collected them as a child. I vividly remember pharmacies in Germany, where I visited when I was young. They had flowers in bottles, lavender for headaches, common sage for sore throats, and rows upon rows of tinctures on their shelves. The pharmacists wore white coats and asked questions. They were kind and placed an extra packet of white tissues in every bag, just in case.

When I was 18, my mother died. I think the helplessness I felt affected me in more ways than one. I wasn't prepared for death, or for life. My body knew what to do: I cried, I froze, and then I ran until I could cry and run no more; then I slept. I share this with you for I have been lost in pain and found a path and chose to help others find theirs, with plants as a guide.

We all have our burdens to carry, some more visible than others, with mixed outcomes, depending on the path we have chosen to take or the support we have. Sometimes we feel out of our depth, at breaking point, lost, not knowing what to do or where to go. I travelled and found huge comfort in plants, nature, and the people I met on my journeys. I found that it was the healing plants, time, and the kindness of others that offered me healing solutions. My pharmacy is world-wide, not exclusive or accessed through white coats "just in case you need it"; it is encapsulated and rooted in nature and, if stored well, is accessible throughout the year.

Hungry to learn about plants, I started working for Neal's Yard Remedies. Unlike a health shop, it was a natural dispensary, with creams and tinctures to make you feel good. The aroma from the blue bottles was familiar, bringing back vivid memories of my childhood. The bell chimed and the learning started when the door opened and people

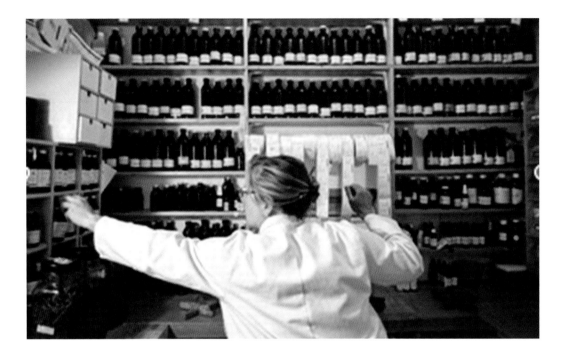

came in, searching for comfort and answers. Some people would bring jars with specimens, in the hope that we could identify the contents; some would even attempt to disrobe in the hope of a physical examination. I learned, I listened; people left with labelled instructions, creams, and bottles of herbs or tiny white pills. Some may have found what they needed. For others, the shop was just part of their signposting so as not to get lost on the journey as they searched for the healing solutions they needed.

Even after completing a degree in phytotherapy (herbal medicine), followed by countless hours of clinical practice, I know that it was the shop and its customers that trained me to think on the spot. I would go home and research the questions that had been raised during the day. Eventually, I could almost hear a ringing sound alerting me to help find among the rows upon rows of bottles and dried herbs the ones that would work best. I would pluck the brown medicine bottles off the shelf like plucking the strings of a harp, ponder and listen, replacing one in favour of another, information flooding my brain. I know this feeling well: my music is the pouring of the liquid, the clinking of glass, the varying pitches of the different measuring cylinders, the stirring and stickiness of the cream.

Knowing which multifaceted liquid will perform its optimum functions in the body when taken in one form or another is like hitting a note in tune with the others. I know that what feels to me like instinct in identifying the correct procedures to follow is actually based on the knowledge drawn from years of study, poring over countless papers and books, and extensive experience of treating my patients.

The plants in the shop had common names, yet for me the Latin classifications held more meaning: "*Leonurus cardiaca*" rolls off my tongue like a musical spell. I also appreciate that using Latin has helped practitioners gain insights across borders and throughout time. However, the shop floor also reminds me to connect in a language we all understand: to keep it simple, so clients don't feel lost in words.

I am an explorer, a medic, mother, daughter, hunter-and-gatherer of knowledge and plants. So, was it the antler chandelier that I inherited from my hunting ancestors that lead me to the trail of Lyme disease? Or the doctor who asked me to join his Lyme team to work collaboratively? Well, he certainly inspired me to travel far to Lyme lectures and research across the world – but no: it was just one person who needed help in unravelling the patterns in symptoms, making connections others may have missed; one single client who tested everything I had learned and prompted me to keep learning and to find answers.

Maybe I was primed at a young age by those detective films and medical mysteries I watched with my grandma now playing out in real life: measurements have consequences. Decades of investigation, clinical practice, differential diagnoses, and materia medica have helped shape my understanding of why people get ill and what plants can help.

At my clinic in Brighton I often hear patients reporting feeling lost, unsure how to proceed. Many of the answers are buried deep. My clients come to me from all walks of life – sometimes I feel as if they are attracted to me the way I am attracted to plants and nature's healing medicine.

I know from my clients that within days of being bitten by a tick, there is a deep feeling of confusion, of being shipwrecked, lost at sea, desperate for a rock to hold on to. Some lucky people have their symptoms recognised by the medical profession, and appropriate treatment is given. Some, however, slip through the net, and, cold, tired, and lonely, they call out for help.

They come to me exhausted, battered by the waves of symptoms, and unhappy with the changing options of help, like tides. Washed up, they hardly recognise themselves, but I recognise their need for a different perspective, a good diet, and herbal medicine.

Together we try to make sense of what has happened, and with the help of plants we find the way forward.

I had a busy client, a doctor, who was referred to me by one of his patients. After consultation, one of my suggestions was to take Japanese knotweed. It so happened that this very invasive plant had recently been removed from the doctor's garden. However, he subsequently reported seeing the plant flourish – and even waving at him in the wind – from his neighbour's garden! Following our consultation, he told me he felt as if the plant had been trying to persuade him to use it, or at least investigate what medicinal properties it might offer. If you are reading this page, you too have been nudged into learning about plants and the many uses a single plant can hold.

Another client, after the second treatment, said, "Still feel on top of the world – you've done things medical professionals have not managed in eleven years!" My hope is that through reading this book you too will be helped in your encounter with Lyme disease.

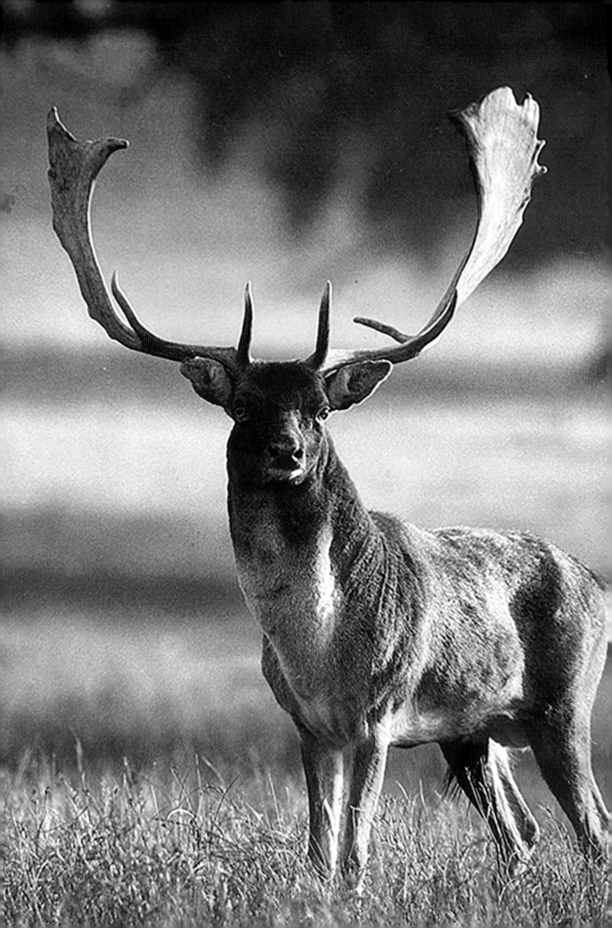

1

What is Lyme disease?

> By 2050, 55.7 million people (12% of the population) in the USA and 134.9 million people (17% of the population) in Europe will have been infected with Lyme disease.[1]

Borreliosis – widely known as Lyme disease – is a bacterial infection, spread to humans by infected ticks. Ticks are tiny arachnids (the size of a sesame seed when young), found in long grass or woodland areas; they feed on the blood of mammals such as deer, mice, rats, cats, and dogs, as well as humans. Tick bites often go unnoticed, unlike those of their relatives – the scorpion or the tarantula, to which one has an immediate reaction even when just hearing their names.

Experience of a woman bitten by a tick

"Being bitten by a tick, I was confused as to what had just happened, but I could not see anything. It was some time later that I looked again, as my ankle was hurting, and then I saw what looked like a tiny black speck of dirt, suctioned onto my ankle, which I removed incorrectly and with great difficulty. I became unwell approximately 12 hours later and then I developed a perfect circular rash around the puncture wound, with slight bruising and reddening, which appeared to be spreading. I am unsure how many days/weeks later it was when I became very unwell, feverish, aching, and feeling like I was losing consciousness. It was then that I was diagnosed by the GP (Dr 1), from my symptoms and the rash.

I panicked when I noticed the rash expanding. I went to a pharmacist, who gave me a steroid cream and said, 'that's a normal reaction to an insect bite'. I phoned NHS 111, who urged me to go to A&E immediately to get the head removed. The two doctors (Dr 2, Dr 3) who saw me couldn't tell if I had Lyme disease or cellulitis and told me to 'wait and see'. Finally another doctor (Dr 4) said 'not to mess about as the consequences of Lyme disease were worse than the antibiotics', so I was prescribed doxy[cycline] for three weeks."

Ticks can be very small and their bite is not painful, so you may not realise you have one attached to your skin. However, there is a higher risk of becoming infected if the tick remains attached to your skin for more than 24 hours.

The common cause of Lyme disease in Europe and North America is the *Borrelia burgdorferi* bacterium, which is passed to humans through the bite of a tick. There are several other Borrelia species that cause

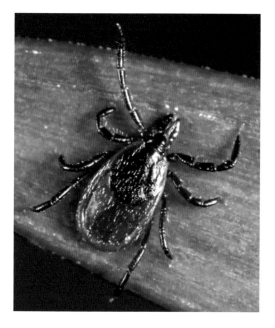

the disease, including *B. afzelii* and *B. garinii*. Another species, *B. miyamotoi*, causes a disease similar to Lyme. Even though it is thought that Lyme disease has been around for hundreds of years, it was only in the 1970s, in Lyme, Connecticut, that it was first recognised and named. It was linked to cases of arthritis in adults and children who also had other puzzling symptoms of what came to be known as Lyme disease.

Borrelia is a spirochete bacterium that infects ticks; it has many species, all behaving like parasites, which explains why antiparasitic herbs like black walnut or berberine-containing plants are often used in treatment. The screw-shaped spirochetes begin to break down collagen in the body and attach to the vascular endothelial cell surface, stimulating flagellin (a protein that all bacteria contain), which activates the release of the NF-κB, a protein that is important for cell survival. This causes an inflammatory and immune response, so herbs like red sage (*Salvia miltiorrhiza*), cordyceps (*Ophiocordyceps sinensis*), and cat's claw (*Uncaria tomentosa*) are often combined, as they are potent NF-κB inhibitors.

Transmission

» Every year, over 232,125 new cases of Lyme disease are reported in Europe[2] – that is, 350 cases per 100,000 people a year. Lyme disease is spreading rapidly throughout Europe and northeast Asia.[3]

» As the life cycle of ticks is strongly influenced by temperature, climate change will increase the range of suitable habitats for them to survive in.

» Estimates of the number of people tested and treated for Lyme disease, based on US insurance claims between 2010 and 2018, are approximately 476,000 a year.[4]

There is a growing incidence of Lyme disease due to the increase in the number of people travelling and to change in habits of the vector – the tick. Lyme disease is a year-round problem, but it is more common during spring and summer, when the ticks are active and feed. When an infected tick bites, the saliva produces anticoagulant compounds that deactivate the inflammatory response you would normally get with an insect bite. Pain signals and itching of the skin are dampened, allowing the tick to continue to feed. If it remains on the skin for several days it will swell to more than twice its size. Depending on the tick's development and the length of time the tick is left on the skin, its saliva can release a specific protein that can interfere with the immune response as it feeds.

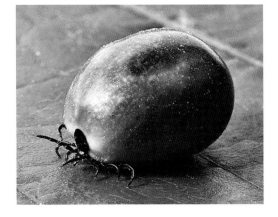

"Initially I thought nothing of the bite that I had in France or the circle that formed around it. It looked a bit odd, unlike any other bite that I'd had, but it didn't itch and wasn't painful so I ignored it and it eventually went away. I had some flu-like symptoms, but nothing severe, so I ignored them as well. It was only a few years later that I saw a picture of an erythema migrans rash and realised that mine had looked exactly the same. By this time I had had a couple of years of bizarre and disabling symptoms, including chronic vertigo/dizziness, extreme fatigue (to the point where I was almost bed-bound for a few months), tingling in my legs, brain fog, confusion, poor memory, skin rashes and migraines. By this point I'd had to take medical retirement from work. Once I saw the picture and found out more about Lyme disease, I set about trying to find a Lyme-literate doctor."

A tick can usually live for 2–3 years and can carry multiple microbes. If the tick acquires a co-infection such as Babesia, a parasite that infects red blood cells in humans, this may have the added benefit for the tick of creating a type of antifreeze compound that stops the tick freezing when the weather gets cold, thus increasing the period over which it is active.

It is estimated that a tick can carry 120 different species of bacteria. If it bites an animal infected with *B. burgdorferi* bacteria, the tick can in turn become infected and can transfer this and other infections (through its "dirty needle") onto humans when it bites them and feeds on their blood.

Once you are infected, the *B. burgdorferi* bacteria move slowly through your skin into your blood and lymphatic system. The latter, which is made up of a series of vessels (channels) and glands (lymph nodes), helps fight infection. Spirochetes move into collagenous tissues; in neuroborreliosis (infection of the nervous system by Borrelia), spirochetes are often present in both the central nervous system and the aqueous humour of the eye within days, which is why infected people often complain of floaters or blurred vision.

"It's like water is trickling down my face, a crawling sensation all the time."

There is no evidence of person-to-person transmission of Lyme disease. Spread from mother to foetus is possible though rare, but with appropriate antibiotic treatment there is no increased risk of adverse birth outcomes.

The three stages of Lyme disease

Stage 1
Early reaction to the local skin infection

A reaction can take as little as 16 hours to appear, or earlier if viral infectious agents have also been transmitted. Symptoms can develop at any time between 3 and 30 days after being bitten by an infected tick.

Bull's-eye rash

The defining symptom of Lyme disease is the appearance of a circular red rash, called erythema migrans. If you see this rash, contact your GP immediately for antibiotics.

The rash is usually a single circular red mark that spreads outwards slowly over several days. The circle gets bigger and bigger, from the size of a dot to at least 5 cm or even larger, with the centre of the circle being where the tick bite occurred. As it spreads outwards, a paler area of skin emerges in the inner part of the circle. This is why the rash is often called a "bull's-eye" rash. It can be mistaken for ringworm.

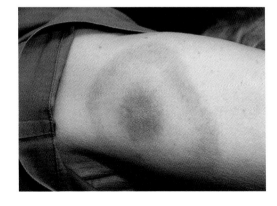

Recognising the rash is helpful in getting a positive diagnosis and early treatment. If Lyme disease is diagnosed early and antibiotic treatment is given within 4 weeks, then the treatment has a higher success rate, thus reducing further complications and cost associated with the disease.[5]

However, the rash is not that common and may occur in only 15–25% of those bitten.

Doctors' varied reactions to a tick bite

"The lack of being taken seriously by the medical profession was stressful. It took me four attempts before they accepted that the slowly expanding but 'atypical' rash at the back of my knee could be an indication of Lymes."

"The GP was confident in his diagnosis, and I remember him saying that there was no point in testing my blood, as it did not always show."

Stage 2
Early spread of infection

"Initially tick bite, rash, known Lyme area. Developed into massive fatigue, pain, aversion to light and sound and profound crankiness. Long-term same symptoms, but less over time."

Builder: "Initially undiagnosed, things were just going downhill. I knew something was wrong. My day looked like: Get up get the kids to school, rest. Go to work, find somewhere to rest/lie down at work (anywhere – it could be on a scaffold, in a cupboard, on a board). Work and come home for lunch. Lie down. Work, rest, get the kids home, rest, fix meal, rest, kids to bed, sleep. My mental state was bad. Bad weird. Someone saying hello could feel like an assault. As I said, weird. Light and sound sensitivities. Diagnosis and treatment with antibiotics provided quick relief from symptoms, but it never lasted, symptoms always returned."

"After having an initial diagnosis I was not worried, after all I had been given antibiotics and it was dealt with, or so I thought. I thought I had been treated and did not think about it again until several years later. After being so unwell over time, it was a gradual realisation, after joining the dots, that a Lyme infection could be the cause of all my bizarre and chronic symptoms."

Symptoms may develop in untreated people weeks or even months after the bite. "Disseminated disease" means that it is spread around the body, away from the site of the original infection. Symptoms are variable but can include one or more of the problems below.

Muscle and joint problems

Joint problems are common and can occur in one or more joints, but most commonly the knee joint. The severity of joint problems can range from episodes of mild pain to severe inflammation (arthritis) causing a lot of pain and weakness. Episodes of joint inflammation last, on average, three months; they may last longer if there is a pre-exiting weakness.

Nerve and brain problems

Nerve inflammation (neuroborreliosis), particularly of the nerves around the face, may develop. (Bell's palsy) This may cause the nerves to stop working, resulting in facial weakness. Inflammation of the tissues around the brain (meningitis) and inflammation of the brain (encephalitis) may follow.

Heart problems

Inflammation of the heart (myocarditis), as well as other heart problems, may develop, giving rise to symptoms such as dizziness, breathlessness, chest pain, and a feeling of the heart beating in a fast, irregular way (palpitations).

Skin problems

Several areas of the skin (not where the tick bite occurred) may develop a rash similar to erythema migrans. These "secondary" rashes tend to be smaller than the original Stage-1 rash and to fade within 3–4 weeks. Occasionally, blue-red nodules called lymphocytomas may develop on the skin, particularly on earlobes and nipples.

Other symptoms

In some rare instances, other organs, such as the eyes, kidneys, and liver, are affected.

Stage 3
Persistent (chronic) Lyme disease

Chronic Lyme disease may appear months or years after infection. It may develop after a period of not having any symptoms. A whole range of symptoms has been described, including chronic joint inflammation, facial palsy with neuropathy, issues with nerves, brain, and heart. Brain problems may include confusion, inability to concentrate, as well as impaired memory, mood, personality, and balance. There may be tiredness and joint pains – called "post-Lyme syndrome" – with symptoms similar to fibromyalgia or chronic fatigue syndrome. Other complications can cause heart rhythm abnormalities and irregularities.

Further complications

A tick can harbour over 120 different microbes. Screening for these and for co-infections will help identify the microbes and other health issues, thus improving your treatment plan and outcome.[6]

Immune suppression as a result of Lyme disease can cause persistent infections or reactivate opportunist infections that often target the site of the body where there is a weakness and amplify it.

As a multisystem illness, Lyme disease can affect and put a strain on all organs. Symptoms can vary, and different people can react differently to the disease and the treatment given. Your past medical history and health can help the practitioner to identify what your achievable goals are.

> "Dental hygiene: my gums and teeth did not feel well with Lyme, I think just due to overall poor health. I eventually had a tooth removed that was irritating, and that, strangely, seem to lead to slight improvement with the Lyme symptoms. Of the latter, I would say an anti-parasitic was of most benefit."

Antiparasitic herbal treatment, combined with a detox, can have some amazing results in reducing symptoms and improving overall health.

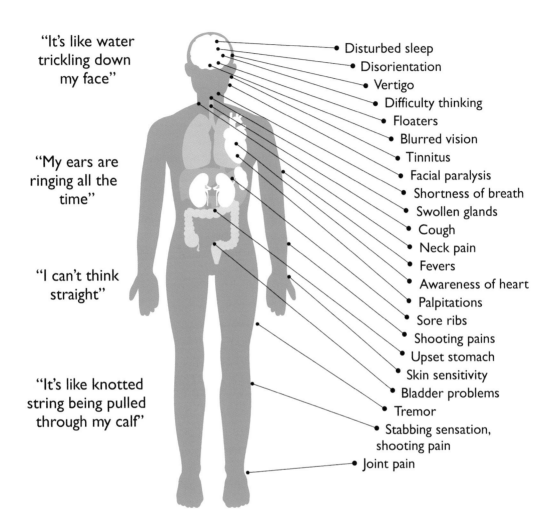

"It's like water trickling down my face"

"My ears are ringing all the time"

"I can't think straight"

"It's like knotted string being pulled through my calf"

- Disturbed sleep
- Disorientation
- Vertigo
- Difficulty thinking
- Floaters
- Blurred vision
- Tinnitus
- Facial paralysis
- Shortness of breath
- Swollen glands
- Cough
- Neck pain
- Fevers
- Awareness of heart
- Palpitations
- Sore ribs
- Shooting pains
- Upset stomach
- Skin sensitivity
- Bladder problems
- Tremor
- Stabbing sensation, shooting pain
- Joint pain

HERBS

- Black walnut
- Cat's claw
- Chinese skullcap
- Ghanaian quinine

- Japanese knotweed
- Siberian ginseng
- Rock rose
- Sweet wormwood

Challenges we face

1. Reducing burden on body
2. Becoming resilient to pathogens
3. Repairing, restoring
4. Reconnecting

BODY MAP 1.1   Symptoms of Lyme disease, the principal herbs in its treatment, and the challenges to be faced.

Oral cavities can contain over 500 different bacteria, which, if left untreated, may lead to surgery, even tooth removal. It appears that spirochetes thrive in dental cavities. Amalgam fillings can harbour *B. burgdorferi* and impede the immune system in detecting pathogens.

> "I was seen by specialists for my mouth pain, who diagnosed nerve damage, trigeminal neuralgia. I am in excruciating oral pain followed by oral cellulitis, sore throat, headaches, neck pain, generalised swelling, overall puffiness, skin rashes, spinal soreness and stiffness, heel pain, and complete exhaustion, weight loss and weight gain (both extreme), sinus problems, digestive upset with severe heartburn and constipation, swollen salivary gland, high blood histamine levels and other raised and deficiency markers detected in my blood, deterioration of sense of smell, chest pain, and breathlessness."

The build-up of heavy metals in the body can add to, or even exacerbate, the many complexities of Lyme disease. Unless treated with detoxification, chelation therapies, and removal of pathogens and toxins, it can adversely affect recovery.

Another complex clinical presentation I often see in my clinic is the recurrence of symptoms of the Epstein-Barr virus (EBV, the cause of mononucleosis/glandular fever). EBV has a picture and clinical presentation similar to Lyme disease: sore throat, fatigue, arthritis myalgia, and fever. There is also a cross-reactivity with antibody tests, which has, in some cases, led to a false-positive of Lyme disease.

Even though EBV is seen as a childhood illness, it can be reactivated at times of stress. Furthermore, infected Lyme cells have been shown to increase replication of EBV, which could be exacerbating the already debilitating symptoms of Lyme disease.

* * *

Between 2015 and 2050 the world's population is predicted to double. Most people want to work later in life, but many are unable to because they are too tired or too sick. The UK Office of National Statistics expect females to be suffering from poor health for their last 20 years and men their last 16.5 years.

So, where Lyme disease is suspected, why not discover things early and prevent or at least warn people of the risk they take so they don't end up in hospital?

Challenges we face when lost in Lyme disease

» *Reducing burden on the body:* by reducing Inflammation and stress triggers, we can further reduce inflammatory symptoms;

» *Becoming resilient to pathogens:* by improving immunity with antimicrobials and using other self-regulating calming activities that can improve resilience;

» *Repairing and restoring:* by improving cognitive function and gut health, stabilising blood sugar, and supporting collagen with herbal remedies and food;

» *Reconnecting with vitality and self:* by meeting our needs through self-care, reflection, and social contact and connection (see STEPS, in chapter 7).

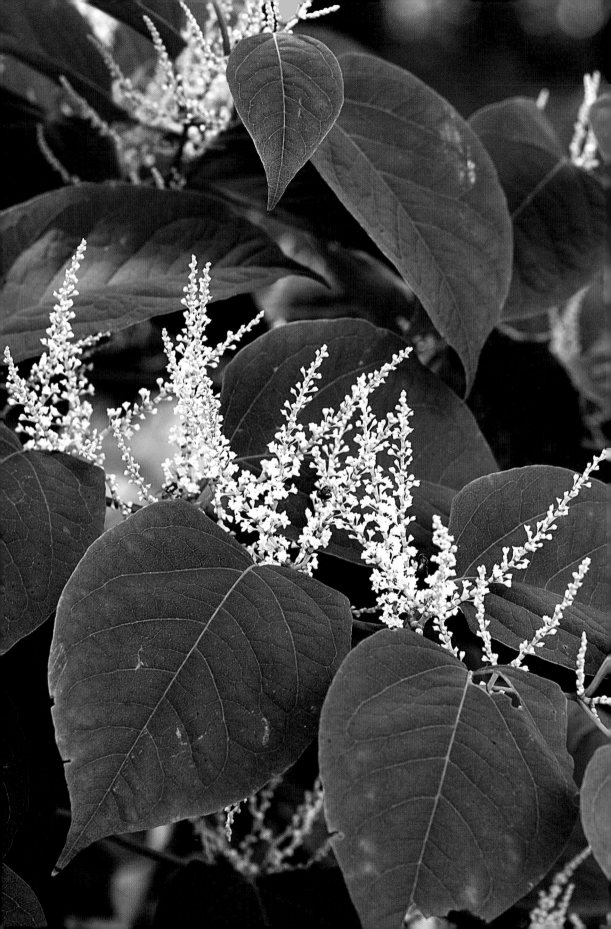

2

Diagnosing and testing for Lyme disease and co-infections

Diagnosing Lyme disease

According to UK NICE guidelines, if you present with a bull's-eye rash, you can be diagnosed and treated for Lyme disease without laboratory testing. The problem is that only some 15% of Lyme sufferers develop the bull's-eye rash; as a result, many people with Lyme disease are not diagnosed correctly and the illness goes undetected, or treatment is given much later, if at all.

In the absence of the typical bull's-eye rash, consideration of the symptoms you are experiencing, coupled with laboratory testing as explained in the next section, can help to guide the diagnosis and treatment. Specific diagnosis of Lyme disease can be difficult, though, as many of the symptoms are similar to those in other conditions. Even if laboratory testing is undergone, a negative result may be false, so it does not exclude a subsequent diagnosis of Lyme disease.

If left untreated, the bacteria that cause Lyme disease can disrupt the immune system and damage collagen, causing hormonal imbalance and inflammation to joints and the nervous system, thus leading eventually to the typical symptoms of Lyme disease.[1]

Potential symptoms of Lyme disease[2]

All of the following are, potentially, symptoms of Lyme disease:

▷ unexplained fevers, sweats, chills, or flushing
▷ unexplained weight change: loss or gain
▷ fatigue, tiredness
▷ unexplained hair loss
▷ swollen glands
▷ sore throat
▷ testicular pain or pelvic pain
▷ unexplained menstrual irregularity
▷ unexplained milk production and/or breast pain
▷ irritable bladder or bladder dysfunction
▷ sexual dysfunction or loss of libido
▷ upset stomach
▷ change in bowel function: constipation or diarrhoea
▷ chest pain or rib soreness
▷ shortness of breath, cough
▷ heart palpitations, pulse skips, heart block
▷ history of a heart murmur or valve prolapse
▷ joint pain or swelling
▷ stiffness of the joints, neck, or back
▷ muscle pain or cramps
▷ twitching of the face or other muscles
▷ headaches
▷ neck aches, neck stiffness
▷ tingling, numbness, burning, or stabbing sensations
▷ facial paralysis (Bell's palsy)
▷ eyes/vision: double, blurry
▷ ears/hearing: buzzing, ringing, ear pain
▷ increased motion sickness, vertigo
▷ lightheadedness, wooziness, poor balance, difficulty walking
▷ tremors
▷ confusion, difficulty thinking
▷ difficulty with concentration or reading
▷ forgetfulness, poor short-term memory
▷ disorientation: getting lost, going to the wrong places
▷ difficulty with speech or writing
▷ mood swings, irritability, depression
▷ disturbed sleep – too much or too little, or early awakening
▷ exaggerated symptoms or worse hangover from alcohol.

Be aware, though, that these may also be symptoms of something other than Lyme disease.

Testing for Lyme disease

"Happy to receive a positive test, it was good to know I wasn't going mad!"

There are various ways of testing for *Borrelia burgdorferi* – the pathogen underlying Lyme disease – and its co-infections. These primarily involve the humoral system (i.e., blood and extracellular fluid) or the cellular system (i.e., cells themselves).

The humoral system: antibody testing

Most Lyme disease tests are designed to detect antibodies made by the body's immune system in response to an infection. These antibodies can take several weeks to develop, so people may test negative if infected only recently.

Conventional antibody testing

Antibody testing, often called serology, addresses the B-cell (a type of white blood cell) response. This usually consists of IgG (Immunoglobulin G) and IgM (Immunoglobulin M). IgM is the first antibody the body makes when it fights a new infection; in most cases, however, it is no longer detectable a few weeks after the original infection.[3] IgG takes time to form after an infection – up to 2 months.[4] However, even if IgG antibodies are detected, conventional medicine will generally dismiss these as a sign of past infection, as IgG antibodies are immune messengers that persist, often for several years, to protect against future infection.

Conventional testing for Lyme disease generally applies the system recommended by the US Centers for Disease Control and Prevention (CDC) in two tiers: an initial test, called "ELISA", determining IgG and

IgM levels, followed, if positive or equivocal, by an IgM and IgG "Western blot" (also called "Immunoblot"), a more specific test. A 2016 meta-analysis of Lyme test accuracy concluded that 46% of cases are being missed with ELISAs and not even being referred for the confirmatory Western blot, where a further 37.5% on average remain undetected.[5]

These results lend support to the conclusion to the effect that "FDA-cleared commercial serological testing for Lyme disease is inadequate for the diagnosis of the disease".[6,7]

The issues mentioned at the outset – relating to when these antibodies, IgM and IgG, are or are no longer detectable during the course of the infection and what they are taken to signify – conventionally mean that this two-tier testing approach is generally of limited use in chronic cases.[8]

More advanced applications of antibody testing

More sophisticated methods and modes of interpretation can still derive benefit from antibody testing for Lyme disease. A multiplex test called TickPlex, developed in Finland and available in Germany, screens for various antigens of Borrelia and in particular the intracellular "round body" or cyst form that the spirochete (i.e., the Borrelia pathogen) forms when it goes into hiding in the tissues: this intracellular "persister" causes the formation of antibodies.[9] While also determining IgG and IgM levels, this technique is very sensitive and gives exact levels. In this way, therapists can identify more easily whether a result is likely to be a continuing infection or reactivation. Many Lyme-literate doctors (LLMDs) have long used the rule of thumb that an IgG four to five times higher than the upper reference range may well be an ongoing or reactivated infection. And the intracellular round-body/cyst form (intracellular persister form) can exhibit a persistent IgM against "round bodies" – that is, be detected even if the infection is chronic, which is missed in conventional ELISA and Western blot analyses.

The cellular system: T-cell immunity

A technique for testing the other arm of the immune system – that is, cellular T-cell immunity – is called ELISpot (enzyme-linked immunospot assay).[10] T-lymphocytes are only present during an active infection and can therefore be used as a marker to reflect a current infection, whether chronic or recent.

The ELISpot is highly sensitive. With detection levels that can be as low as 1 cell in 100,000, it is one of the most sensitive cellular assays available.[11] This technique has long been used in Germany to quantify T-cells that secrete signature proteins (such as a given cytokine) against a specific antigen. The Borrelia ELISpot evaluates the number of spot-forming units using a stimulation index (SI) based on IGRA (Interferon Gamma Release Assay), thus providing a measurement of B. burgdorferi-sensitive T-cells in the blood. A result of 0–1 is negative, over 1 is borderline, 2–3 is weak positive, and greater than 3 is positive. This is also a helpful tool for monitoring treatment progression, as the T-cellular immune response should vanish after 4–8 weeks of an effective therapeutic strategy.

Polymerase chain reaction (PCR) test

A Borrelia PCR test is an amplified nucleic acid assay intended to detect DNA sequences from various genes specific to the pathogen.[12] This is not the first test of choice, as these gene fragments are not always easily detectable in the blood of those with Lyme disease.

Testing for co-infections

There are multiple co-infections of Lyme disease: it rarely occurs alone. As mentioned earlier, the "dirty needle" of a tick or other biting arthropod may well transfer other infections. Many infections – such as viruses – can arise as opportunistic infections when the immune system is suppressed (as it can be with Lyme disease).

Examples of co-infections that can be tested for, using both ELISpot and antibody testing, are:

▷ Anaplasma/Ehrlichia
▷ Babesia
▷ Bartonella
▷ Borrelia miyamotoi
▷ Chlamydia
▷ Cytomegalovirus (CMV)
▷ Enteroviruses Coxsackie and Echovirus

> Epstein–Barr virus (EBV)
> Herpes simplex virus (HSV 1/2)
> Human herpes virus (HHV–6, –7, and –8)
> Mycoplasma
> Rickettsia
> SARS-CoV–2
> Varicella-zoster virus (VZV)
> Yersinia enterocolitica bacteria

It is possible to determine which specific co-infection to test for by using the specialised checklists that the labs usually supply, always taking into consideration your full history and symptoms.

Immunoglobulin A

The antibody IgA (Immunoglobulin A) for many of the above infections exists as a test (though rarely in the United Kingdom) mostly at overseas laboratories such as ArminLabs in Germany. This is a very useful antibody, as an IgA (to the Coxsackie virus, for example) tends to persist along the mucosal membranes. This generally signifies an ongoing infection, even if chronic.[13]

CD57 marker

The CD57 marker is present on natural killer (NK) cells and T lymphocytes and was at one point thought to be an important indicator for chronic Lyme diagnosis. However, some practitioners find this a misleading indicator for Lyme disease as a stand-alone test, because MS, systemic lupus, rheumatoid arthritis, HIV, herpes, as well as chronic Lyme patients all often show a low CD57 count (less than 100 CD57 cells/μl).

Many of my clients with Lyme disease have a low CD57 count (around 60), but they also often have a compromised immune system with a history of viral infections, such as herpes. A rise in CD57 can indicate that treatment is working. It is important to recognise that children will also present with a low CD57, as their immune systems are not yet fully formed.

A rise in CD57 can indicate that treatment is working.

* * *

Even though lab tests for initial screening can be important here, they can also change and are not always 100% reliable. Some laboratories use questionnaires and other forms as a tool to work out which test would be appropriate.

Tests and clinical findings can be difficult to interpret; however, labs and clinics may be helpful in explaining results or discoveries. It is worth bearing in mind that more than one test may be needed, for co-infections, hormonal abnormalities, mineral deficiencies, stool samples abnormalities, food allergies or sensitivities, autoimmune overlaps, heavy-metal burdens and toxins, genetic detoxification problems, as well as cortisol and insomnia problems. Some tests may be available from the local health care provider, but others may be more difficult to obtain; it is, however, important to test the function of the liver, heart, and kidneys, especially if antibiotics have been or are being taken.

A holistic health care provider looks at the whole person, not just the symptoms or test results.

> "A positive ELISA test came back, but the Western blot must have been negative, as the overall result came back negative. I was never given what bandings on the Western blot reacted. Infectious Disease retested me, and the result was described to me as equivocal, so it is not a definite positive, but it is not negative either."

Do not rely on tests alone

Lyme can inhibit the immune system, giving rise to false-negative antibody tests. A recent paper analysed cases diagnosed with Lyme disease in a London hospital.[14] It reported that 11 people who had a negative ELISA screening test were thought by their doctors to have Lyme disease. Their blood was therefore sent for a Western blot despite the negative ELISA. Of these 11, 6 had a positive Western blot.

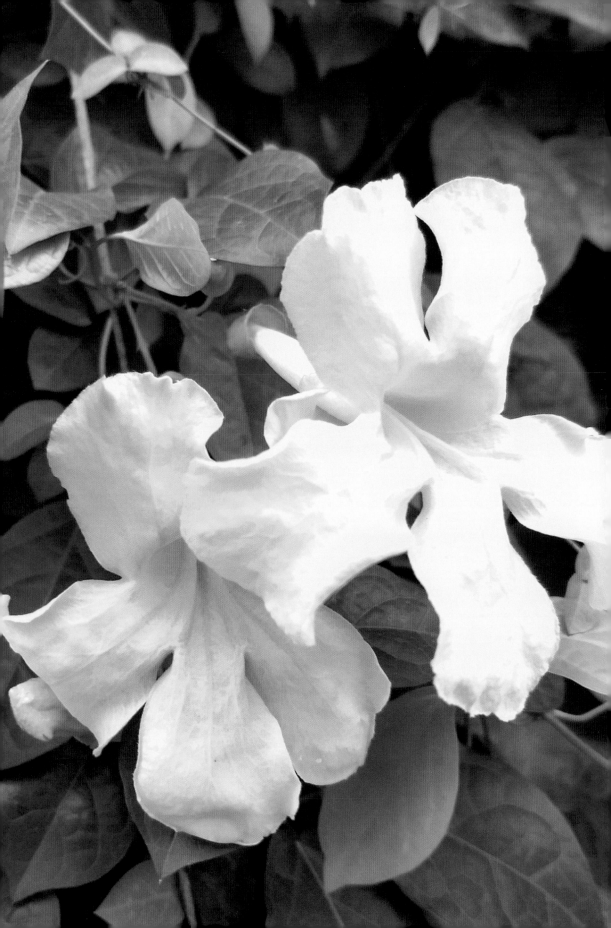

3

Minimising risk, precautions, and differential diagnosis

How common is Lyme disease?

Lyme disease is the most common tick-borne infectious disease in the United Kingdom, Europe, and North America.

Public Health England reports that in the United Kingdom there are between 2,000 and 3,000 cases a year confirmed by a positive test, and that about 15% of these confirmed infections are acquired when travelling outside the UK. Scotland has 27% of all UK cases of Lyme disease.

However, as Lyme disease has many symptoms, is difficult to diagnose, and testing for it can be unreliable, it is likely that at least 8,000 people in the United Kingdom have Lyme disease – at least three to four times more than previously thought. Some believe that even that figure is an underestimation.

As mentioned in chapter 1, tens of thousands of cases of Lyme disease are reported in the United States every year.

Groups most at risk

The majority of tick bites happen from spring to autumn, when people are most likely to take part in outdoor activities. Because areas such as woodland and heath are inhabited by tick-carrying animals such as deer and mice, the groups most at risk of getting Lyme disease are those who work or take part in activities in these areas. For example:

- dog walkers and owners
- hikers
- campers
- plant gatherers
- foragers
- farmers
- gamekeepers
- forestry workers
- military personnel

"I was bitten by a tick while in the New Forest. The tick had been attached for at least 72 hours.

I began feeling unwell, exhausted, so I spoke to my doctor, who prescribed doxy[cycline], but I couldn't tolerate this so was changed to amoxicillin for 3 weeks. In the break between anti-biotics, I began experiencing sensitivity to light, trouble focusing eyes. Had two optician appointments, and there was nothing wrong with my eyes. I then started having weakness and numb-ness in legs and hands. I also had facial paralysis; I was started on steroids for 10 days, and the paralysis cleared up. I had constant pain in my face and nausea. I'd gone from a fit healthy 35-year-old to feeling weak and exhausted every day and I am still having eye issues.

I started taking herbs, and within one month all symptoms all cleared.

I feel normal again, back to my old self. I can't believe it, I thought it would never clear."

If you do find a tick on you, put it in a small container such as a bottle or plastic bag, Label the container with your name, the date, the location of the tick bite, and how long the tick was attached. You can then take the tick to a testing facility or your healthcare provider to be tested for diseases.

Preventing Lyme disease

Currently, there is no approved vaccine to prevent Lyme disease. In 1998, a vaccine was introduced in America, but the manufacturer withdrew it in 2002 citing insufficient consumer demand. However, at least two vaccines are under early stages of clinical trial in the United States.[1]

Precautions

If you do find a tick on your (or someone else's) skin, remove it carefully by twisting it off with a tick remover. It is essential that the mouth parts are removed in addition to the body. A paste created by mixing slippery elm or clay with some andrographis tincture can be used to cover the bite to help draw out any toxins. Removal of an attached tick within the first 24 hours will usually prevent an infection.

Put the tick in a Ziploc bag or other container in the freezer, so it can, if necessary, be sent off and tested.

Precautions to help prevent Lyme disease

» Wear a long-sleeved shirt.
» Tuck your trousers into long socks.
» Use insect repellent.
» Avoid long grass, and stay on the path.
» Check yourself for ticks.
» Check your children and pets for ticks.

If you discover a rash, develop feverish symptoms, or feel unwell, consult your doctor. Take photos of the rash, then mark it with a pen to check whether it is growing.

As a preventative measure in high-risk areas during tick season (May–September), or all year round if you work outdoors, the noted herbalist Stephen Buhner recommends taking astragalus, with meals. Astragalus is an immune regulator; it increases the effect of enzymes that activate white blood cells and supports immune function.

For new tick bites, Buhner typically recommends taking astragalus 3,000 mg daily for 30 days and 1,000 mg daily thereafter until symptoms improve. However, if symptoms persist or get worse, stop taking it.[2]

Astragalus is not recommended in chronic Lyme disease.

Differential diagnosis

Many practitioners refer to Lyme disease as the great imitator, as Lyme disease and its co-infections can mimic many illnesses. It may not be the only medical condition at play, and life-style choices may also have affected the strength of the immune system. People can feel overwhelmed at times because of the variation in symptoms. One of the ways to pinpoint which illness(es) actually is present is via differential diagnosis, which tests for all potential illnesses, one by one. Richard Horowitz[3] describes this by saying that if you have numerous nails in your foot and you remove one of the nails, your foot may still hurt but you are one step closer to isolating the cause of the pain.

Imitators of Lyme disease

Conversely, some conditions are seen as imitators of Lyme disease. They may also be contributing to the experience of having the disease and therefore still need addressing and treating.

Mineral deficiency or toxicity

Toxic overload can manifest itself in numerous ways: headache, irritability, brain fog, constipation, skin breakouts. When the body is overloaded with toxins from pollutants in its environment, it can cause stress on the liver and kidneys. There may be feelings of tingling or numbness or burning sensations, which may be a neuropathy caused by a genetic or vitamin deficiency (B12, folic acid), heavy metal toxicity (mercury, lead, arsenic), thyroid or hormonal disorder, or immune deficiency. It is also an indication for checking autoimmune markers against the nerves and neurotoxins. Many of these symptoms can be similar to Lyme disease and further contribute to the burden of the parasites and co-infections associated with the disease.

Blood sugar imbalances

Blood sugar imbalances may make you feel tired, have mood swings, have concentration problems, feel dizzy with palpitations, or need a nap soon after lunch. Eating regularly and getting blood checks can easily remedy this.

Allergies and histamine intolerance

Allergies or an increase in histamine may cause symptoms of heart palpitations, increases in inflammation, swollen throat or ankles, bronchiole constriction, headaches, hives, nasal congestion, anxiety, breast tenderness, insomnia and brain fog. In women, there may be hormonal links during certain stages of the menstrual cycle connected to histamine intolerance.

Mast cell disorders

Mast cell activation syndrome is rare but can also cause the body to release chemicals in the body activating a series of inflammatory reactions, in a manner similar to or further complicating a Lyme picture. Mast cell disorders can cause mast cell dysfunction syndrome, which can, in turn, cause a range of symptoms similar to allergies, gut, mood, and skin changes, and muscle and joint pain.

Gut flora disturbances

Gut flora disturbances, such as small intestinal bacterial overgrowth (SIBO) causing an imbalance of gut bacteria or low acid, can contribute to high-histamine depression, anxiety, and immune dysfunction.

Fungal infections

The use of antibiotics and some other medications can cause fungal overgrowth in the body. This can affect the mouth, vagina, and gut. Symptoms can be pain, itchy skin, fatigue, depression, joint pain, sinus and digestive issues. Richard Horowitz describes over two thirds of his patients having signs of chronic persistent disease due to mould toxins.[4]

Stretch-like marks: Bartonella

Lines, or stretch-like marks, can be one of the signs of Bartonella infection. It should be noted, however, that these are not stretch marks, such as those that mothers might develop after pregnancy or teenagers after a sudden growth spurt.

Menopause

Hot flushes, night sweats, insomnia, fatigue, anxiety, mood swings, irritability, and depression can be menopausal and mimic symptoms of Lyme disease.

Babesia

Babesia, a parasitic infection, can often cause symptoms such as day sweats, night sweats, fevers, chills, and air hunger.

PoTS

Postural orthostatic tachycardia syndrome (PoTS) affects blood flow and the nervous system. With this condition, you can feel extremely tired, dizzy, experience neck pain, tremors, and poor cognition. Performing sitting and standing pulse-rate and blood-pressure measurements may help to identify PoTS, as pulse increases and blood pressure can drop 30 bpm.

Chronic fatigue syndrome

Chronic fatigue syndrome (CFS) is a particularly severe form of fatigue and is a complex condition. It has been associated with chronic infection, previous viral infection, and mitochondrial, hormonal, and adrenal dysfunction. With this condition you may also have problems thinking clearly and feel dizzy, depressed, or anxious.

Fibromyalgia

Fibromyalgia is a painful condition that affects 1 in 20 people. It is 7 times more common in women than in men and can cause widespread pain, stiffening of muscles, headaches, brain fog, irritable bowel syndrome (IBS), and fatigue. The cause is unclear. Stress or a change in weather can make it worse. Orthodox medicine tends to prescribe cognitive behavioural therapy (CBT), antidepressants, or painkillers.

Autoimmune disorders

Rheumatoid arthritis, multiple sclerosis (MS), and lupus are all autoimmune disorders, where the immune system sees the body as foreign and attacks it, causing flares of fatigue, muscle pain, and a low fever.

   MS is an immune-related disorder affecting the nervous system. It can cause symptoms similar to those of Lyme disease, such as blurred vision, confusion, burning and stabbing pain, or a crawling sensation or pins and needles in muscles. Lumbar puncture and MRI scan can distinguish this condition from Lyme disease.

Ehlers–Danlos syndrome

Ehlers–Danlos syndrome is a genetic disorder that causes hypermobile joints and can affect connective tissues supporting the bowel, skin, bones, blood vessels, and many other organs and tissues. Defects in connective tissues cause signs and symptoms ranging from mildly loose joints to life-threatening complications. Oesophageal and gastric issues can cause slow transit times and problems around the colon. What can further complicate this picture from a Lyme perspective is that Ehlers–Danlos syndrome is associated with coeliac markers that could further complicate identifying cause and symptoms, especially if gluten is not eliminated from one's diet.[5] Those with Lyme disease and Ehlers–Danlos syndrome often have a high pain threshold, so obvious signposting or support can often be delayed.

Complexity of treatment: snapshots of clients' experiences

Experience of treatment, after visiting A&E for a test in 2009

"I was referred to a Dr (no. 2) privately up North, who prescribed a lot of antibiotics: 2 weeks on doxy[cycline], 2 weeks metronidazole, 2 weeks 1,000 mg three times a day amoxicillin, cycling them with 2 weeks off, then starting again. Did 3 cycles, then had low-dose naltrexone obtained from a pharmacy in Scotland. Then I was referred to a Dr (no. 3) by the Dr (no. 1) in A&E. He liaised with the Dr 2 up north and took more bloods. Dr 3 wasn't too keen on antibiotics and prescribed hydrogen peroxide transfusions intravenously monthly, and a high dose of amoxicillin by the Dr 2 up North, so I took those.

Symptoms: Itching, pain, brain fog, tiredness, joint pain, neck pain, flitting aches, memory issues, bowel and bladder issues, foot pain, heart aches, mental health issue, period issues. Reflux, digestive issues. Weird swellings in fingers.

I continued with Dr 2, drinking oxygenated oils based on the Klinghardt Protocol.[6] I think this seemed to help. I also went to a private hospital who claim to specialise in Lyme disease (didn't find helpful: budget needed insane and very impersonal, in my experience) and have had my blood tested at a German lab, which was showing there is still active disease; this wasn't recognised by the NHS.

Then Dr 2 was struck off, I think."

The question remains, which active disease is causing the problem?

Orthodox medication for an arthritis diagnosis made this patient feel worse.

> "Arthritis, rheumatoid arthritis, or I could 'just' still have Lyme, but no way of knowing. The difficulty of not being able to have a long-term Lyme/co-infections diagnosis is mentally exhausting. Hot yoga and herbs have stopped me getting worse."

This client no longer attends my clinic but she does join us on my long foraging walks, which is, in my eyes, a form of recovery in itself, and she is a great help and inspiration to me and to others.

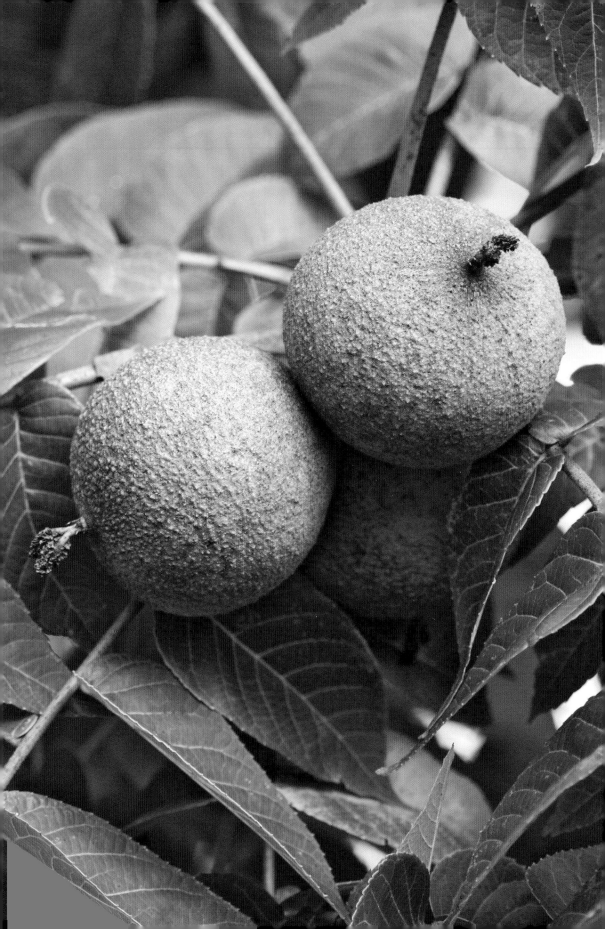

4

Medical treatment and herbal remedies

A common request from my clients is for information about antibiotics. This chapter begins by outlining the antibiotics doctors prescribe for Lyme disease. Some GPs find long-term intravenous antibiotics for treating chronic Lyme disease more successful than tablets, others do not. As with all medication and treatment, there are downsides, and these are also outlined here.

> It is reported by the New England Journal of Medicine, that 10–20% of people continue to suffer from Lyme disease symptoms after antibiotic treatment.[1]

The second part of the chapter discusses in depth how herbal medicine can be effective in reducing some of the risks and side effects associated with taking medications prescribed for Lyme disease. It also then considers natural antibiotics and herbal treatments.

Drug treatment for Lyme disease

"The IV antibiotics got me out of the paralysed situation. Further antibiotics took me so far, but no real improvement. I still had most of my symptoms. Herbal medicine was the turning point for me. Yes, I still have problems even after years of treatment, but you learn that nothing moves fast with treating Lyme disease."

General information on taking antibiotics

If antibiotics are started soon after the tick bite, patients often recover within two or three months. In this acute phase, the Lyme symptoms usually disappear in most, although not all, people. The two drugs most commonly used in the early treatment of Lyme disease are doxycycline (a tetracycline) and amoxicillin (a penicillin).

Antibiotics destroy both beneficial and non-beneficial bacteria in your intestinal tract. The former are essential for proper digestion, detoxification, cognitive function, and your overall health in general. Take antibiotics after the beginning of a meal, once there is some food in your stomach.

Herbal preparations can improve absorption of antibiotics while supporting gut health and aiding nutrient uptake from food.

Replacing the beneficial bacteria is essential, as examined in this and later chapters. If you are on a course of antibiotics, it is worth considering taking probiotics like acidophilus; these must be taken at night, at least one hour before or after any antibiotics. However, probiotics may not always be appropriate, especially in cases of histamine sensitivity.

> Probiotics should not be confused with prebiotics, which are foods that provide nutrients that encourage bacteria essential to health to thrive.

A combination of antibiotics may be prescribed by doctors; this will necessitate monthly blood tests to check liver and kidney function. If taking multiple antibiotics simultaneously causes you stomach issues, take the antibiotics apart from one another, with food. Do not take multimineral supplements or antacids less than one hour before or after antibiotics, as they may interact adversely with them.

Some people feel worse after starting antibiotics or too unwell to continue taking them (see the section below, "Herxheimer reactions"). This could be either part of the healing process or a reaction to the antibiotics, so it is important to speak to your health care provider before making any changes to treatment.

Grapefruit juice and dairy can also interact adversely with antibiotics, so it is best to avoid taking them at the same time. Similarly, if you are using herbal medicine and vitamins, it is important that you inform your practitioner, as these too could interact with the antibiotics.

> "I tried 5 weeks of antibiotics by IV followed by 2 weeks of oral antibiotics, but had to stop as I felt terrible. Sadly I haven't seen a great improvement in symptoms. I think I very much fall into the 'existing health issue' category and my immune system is pretty shot having been ill for 13 years."

Skin rashes, stomach upset, yeast overgrowth, headaches are common side effects reported with antibiotics. They may also cause loose stools, nausea, vomiting, diarrhoea, dizziness, spinning sensations.

> According to Caudwell LymeCo Charity and Lyme Disease UK, February–April 2016, over a third of patients with Lyme disease were not given antibiotics.

It is worth noting that antibiotics may decrease the efficacy of birth control pills, so it would be wise to use additional protection (e.g., condoms) while on antibiotics.

Longer-term treatment

Some clients and doctors feel that treatment for Lyme disease may require a longer course of antibiotics. Yet doctors often have to follow guidelines that indicate short-term use. There are a few GPs who feel that if the symptoms continue after the antibiotics course has finished, there may be a case for intravenous antibiotics. It is important to be clear that antibiotics are not always effective at the later stage of Lyme disease, as the bacteria can change into cyst form, making it harder for the immune system to pick up and identify the bacteria.

Decisions regarding antibiotics can be further complicated by the fact that some people are intolerant of the antibiotics most commonly prescribed for Lyme disease, such as doxycycline, amoxicillin, and cefuroxime. In this case, clarithromycin, macrolides, azithromycin, or erythromycin are used, but these alternatives may have lower efficacy yet still cause side effects.

Types of antibiotics

There are two classes of antibiotics used in the treatment of Lyme disease: *bactericidal* antibiotics, which kill bacteria directly; and *bacteriostatic* antibiotics – such as the tetracyclines – which stop bacteria from growing but do not kill them.

Hydroxychloroquine, although not itself an antibiotic, is also prescribed in the treatment of Lyme disease, as it increases the effectiveness of antibiotics.

Bactericidal antibiotics

Amoxicillin

Amoxicillin is a penicillin-type antibiotic used for general urinary and respiratory infections and for early diagnosed Lyme disease and associated cardiac abnormalities. It is usually taken for 21 days.

Azithromycin and clarithromycin

Azithromycin and clarithromycin are used for bacterial infections, including stomach ulcers caused by *Helicobacter pylori,* as well as for relapsing fever associated with Lyme disease. Regular cardiac check-ups are important, especially if there are symptoms of persistent new muscle pain, as it may affect your heart.

There may possibly be interactions between clarithromycin and prescription medications, so inform your GP of any medication you are taking.

Side effects include new or increased ringing in the ears, hearing problems, nausea, sore tongue, vomiting, difficulty swallowing, diarrhoea, liver toxicity, and pancreatitis.

Intravenous ceftriaxone

Ceftriaxone, which is administered intravenously, is an extremely specialised antibiotic, rare and difficult to get hold of. It has been prescribed by some specialists for chronic Lyme disease affecting the central nervous system or for Lyme carditis. It is provided by specialist clinics, with varying degrees of success.

Tinidazole and metronidazole

Tinidazole (Tindamax) and metronidazole (Flagyl) are antibiotic and antiprotozoal medications. They can cause neuropathy or increase an existing Lyme neuropathy, so if there is any increase in tingling and numbness, stop the medication and contact your doctor.

Avoid ALL alcohol, including mouthwashes or perfumes/colognes containing alcohol. Herbal or alcohol-based tinctures should be decreased if any nausea occurs. Multivitamins with a B-complex, or Methyl Protect and/or vitamin B6 100 mg per day, taken one hour before or after this form of medication, may also help to reduce neuropathic symptoms.

Rifampin

Rifampin inhibits bacteria reproduction and is effective for a number of bacterial conditions such as chlamydia and mycobacteria, which can sometimes cause co-infections in Lyme disease. Rifampin may affect other drug levels in your body. An unexpected side effect is that your urine may turn orange.

Richard Horowitz has found that Rifampin, combined with doxycycline and the leprosy drug dapsone, over an eight-week course is effective in improving symptoms in 98% of patients.[2]

Side effects of Rifampin include headaches, itching, dizziness, flushing, yellow colouring of skin. Your tears may turn orange and may stain contact lenses.

Tetracyclines

The tetracyclines are a class of broad-spectrum antibiotics. Strict sun avoidance is necessary when taking tetracyclines as they can cause photosensitive reactions and sunburn; sun exposure should be limited as far as possible and high SPF sunscreen used on all exposed areas, including lips.

Doxycycline

Doxycycline, one of the tetracyclines, is used to help relieve muscle/joint involvement or diseases affecting the cranial nerves or the peripheral nervous system. It is usually taken for 2–4 weeks.

For many people, doxycycline can cause a tummy upset, and it is not recommended to increase to a higher dose, if necessary, until you feel better and the doxycycline is well tolerated.

In areas where there is a very high risk of a tick bite, a single prophylactic dose of doxycycline may be given.

Minocycline

Minocycline, another tetracycline, is used when there are more cognitive and neurological symptoms in chronic Lyme disease, as it is lipid-soluble and crosses the blood–brain barrier.

Hydroxychloroquine (Plaquenil)

The bark of the cinchona tree has been used for centuries in the treatment of malaria. In the 1820s the alkaloid quinine was extracted from the bark, and purified quinine is still being used today as an antimalarial medication. Modern synthetic versions are chloroquine and hydroxychloroquine, both of which are antimalarials. Hydroxychloroquine is prescribed by rheumatologists for lupus, rheumatoid arthritis, etc. Doctors currently use it for Lyme disease to attack the cystic forms and to increase the effectiveness of antibiotics. It should not be used if there are any visual-field or colour-vision problems.

Herxheimer reactions

"I did not improve but became sicker. On reflection I think it was a Herxheimer reaction, but did not know what a Herx was during that acute phase of illness."

The Herxheimer reaction is a short-term worsening of symptoms and/or co-infections following treatment for an illness. Also known as Herxing, it refers to symptoms that are associated with the body breaking down and getting rid of pathogens as a result of using antibiotics or herbs. It often follows treatment for Lyme disease. Not all people experience a Herxheimer reaction, but some find it incredibly difficult and have to stop treatment. There are also those who welcome symptoms associated with the reaction as a sign that their body is eliminating Lyme disease. Symptoms can last for weeks and can include a worsening of fever, chills, muscle pains, confusion, and headache.

It is important to differentiate between a Herxheimer reaction and an adverse drug reaction. Generally, drug reactions can occur within an hour after initiating antibiotics, while a Herxheimer reaction may not become apparent for 48–72 hours.

The Herxheimer reaction can be severe and may cause a people to stop taking antibiotics or herbs altogether, as it can feel as though you are having the worst hangover ever, with nausea, headaches, chills, increased pain, and a crash in energy. Endotoxins released from the body may overwhelm and create a toxic burden on the system.

The reaction may feel much worse than the treatment. There is no point continuing to kill off spirochetes until this period has passed, although you should not stop taking medication without discussion with your doctor. You can help the body by increasing fluid intake, improving the circulation, and using lymphatic herbs to help the body rid itself of dead bacteria and the overload of the system.

Detoxification may help with the Herxheimer reaction, alongside herbs taken at a low dose and then slowly built up. Avoid fasting, juicing programmes, and saunas, as these increase bacteria die-off and may be too much for you. These will be useful later, however, when you are feeling better; some people may also benefit from infrared saunas.

The following section details herbs, foods, and lifestyle changes that may help alleviate some symptoms by improving elimination channels of detoxification.

Managing Herxheimer reactions

Natural detox aids

Nausea remedies: Teas good for dealing with nausea are chamomile or peppermint tea. Ginger, a circulatory stimulant, is useful for nausea as it calms the digestive system; it can be grated into food or added to tea or taken in the form of one capsule with each meal.

Headache remedies: Helpful herbs include: feverfew, wood betony, kudzu, rosemary, skullcap, valerian, chamomile, and peppermint tea.

Heartburn and indigestion remedies: Slippery elm can reduce discomfort and has the added benefit of being a prebiotic, feeding friendly bacteria in the gut: 1 tablet twice a day, two hours before or after food. You can also mix the powder into water or yoghurt.

Lymphatic support: 50 ml of pressed cleaver juice, or 5–10 ml of tincture of cleaver a day can help with detoxification and the Herxheimer reaction. (Drop dose of poke root, available from a qualified practitioner, may also be of use.)

Kidney cleansing: Enjoy a juice first thing as part of a cleanse, made up of the juice of ¼ lemon, ½ tsp raw honey (optional), 1 tsp organic apple cider vinegar with mother, ¼ tsp bicarb, and half a glass of warm water, or equal part of *Uva ursi*, nettle, and horsetail infusion, tsp 3 x a day.

Sleeping well: to reduce stress levels, try to keep regular eating and sleeping hours, balancing blood sugar levels. Herbs such as chamomile, valerian, passionflower, Jamaican dogwood (*Piscidia*), or jujube (*Zizyphus*) can be of help.

Meditation: Practice slow, deep, diaphragmatic breathing (no more than 10 breaths per minute) with a longer out-breath than in-breath: this enables your brain to calm down and move out of a sympathetic nervous (stressed) state, into a parasympathetic nervous (relaxed) one. Do this at least three times a day for around 15 minutes each time, or whenever you feel yourself getting anxious.

Hyperbaric oxygen or ozone therapy: Some practitioners use different forms of oxygen therapy; this has a wide range of applications, ranging from inactivating cell walls of bacteria and fungi, including spores, and enhancing white blood cells to killing bacteria and promoting absorption of medication into cells. It sometimes provides relief from Herxheimer symptoms, aiding detoxification. Many bacteria, including Borrelia, thrive in a low-oxygen environment. Therapy that floods the organism with oxygen can often provide relief from symptoms of Lyme disease.[3]

Taking additional nutrients: *Quercetin* is a strong antioxidant that is often taken as a supplement to minimise Herxheimer reactions and inflammation. Raised histamine or mast cell activation is common in people with Lyme disease, and reducing these levels can be of significant benefit. Quercetin is found in vegetables, grains, tea, and red wine. Its absorption is increased when taken with bromelain – an enzyme found in pineapples. Take 500 mg/day of quercetin with 100 mg of bromelain and 500 mg of vitamin C.

Glutathione (available as a supplement, liposomal glutathione), an antioxidant, is important for the detoxification of heavy metals and cellular repair after damage. Treating zinc and vitamin B6 deficiencies (e.g., with supplements) increases glutathione, which is particularly helpful in reducing Herxheimer reactions, inflammation of the liver, and brain fog and for restoring cognitive function. (Take 500 mg liposomal glutathione once or twice a day.)

Coping with toxins

In my experience, only a minority of people have any concept of how debilitating a toxin load and its consequential damage can be. It is an underestimation to say this fight is a challenge, as it is so much more.

Some people I see have been sick for a long time and may have many underlying conditions contributing to their ill health.

> "At the age of 58, I suddenly developed debilitating migraines, which, at their worst, could last for three days, and I was lucky to get two weeks without one. Apart from the terrible physical pain and nausea, there was also a psychological effect: I could hardly go out. Holidays, social events, even doctors' appointments were marred with the thought, "Am I going to be okay?" My GP could only offer me medication once the migraine had started and had no idea as to why they were occurring. I spent years having acupuncture, homeopathy, Chinese herbs, all of which had some effect, but nothing like a cure.
>
> I made an appointment with a medical herbalist as a last resort, because I had tried everything else. For the first time in four years, I went three months without a migraine, then nine months, with only two very mild headaches.
>
> I had started to think that I would have to live with migraines forever – now I don't."

The following are a number of herbal and other therapies that can aid detoxification.

Charcoal: Derived from carbonised organic materials, such as coconut shells or bamboo. It has a history of effective affordable short-term use, absorbing and binding toxins in food poisoning and other digestive complaints. It is used in the treatment of mould or antifungal protocols and is particularly helpful where there is gas, bloating, or headaches from toxic overload. Binders should be taken some time before or after food, so they do not affect mineral absorption. Dose can vary, depending on the individual: 1,000–1,500 mg (2–3 capsules) twice daily with water, or once at night. (*Note:* Highly sensitised people with a histamine or mast cell activation syndrome may need a specialised histamine protocol, with diet, botanical and prescription antihistamines, before binders can be used.)

Chlorella: Has the powerful detoxifying ability to bind to toxins and prevent them from being reabsorbed in the digestive tract. Take 1–5 g a day before meals, mixed into water or pomegranate juice, or 1 tsp to 1 tbsp of tincture per day.

Milk thistle: Protects the liver from toxins, drugs, alcohol, and viruses and helps to repair liver damage. It promotes the secretion of bile from the gallbladder, increasing bowel movements and removing stagnation from the liver, aiding detoxification.

Powdered Zeolite: Powder from volcanic rock is used to help bind toxins that are released from heavy metals or the die-off of pathogens such as viruses, bacteria, fungi, and mould. Binders like Zeolite and charcoal bind toxins, reducing diarrhoea and hangover-type symptoms, increasing bowel movements, and removing unwanted toxins.[4]

Sarsaparilla: Helps to bind and remove toxins released from bacteria cell membranes. It also helps to reduce inflammation, protects the body from the toxins, and increases liver and energy function in the body. It can be taken as a tincture or a tea.

Relax while you gently detox!

Epsom salts (magnesium sulphate): These bath salts can help to relieve the stress that comes with and causes adrenal fatigue. Magnesium acts as a muscle relaxer, and the sulfur increases bile production in the liver, enabling the elimination of toxins, particularly those stored in fats. Magnesium aids in the elimination of toxins from the pores, easing muscle pain. Two handfuls of Epsom salts added to the bath, soak for 15 minutes up to three times a week. Drink water to help with your detox. Be sure you are rehydrated before taking a detox bath.

Dry-brush your body: To enhance the effect of the bath, dry-brush your entire body before you step into the bathtub. This helps to open the pores and stimulate the lymphatic system.

Exercise: Increases glutathione levels, thereby helping to boost the immune system, improve detoxification, and enhance the body's own antioxidant defences. Start slowly, building up to 30 minutes a day of vigorous aerobic exercise like swimming, walking or jogging, hot yoga, or playing various sports. Strength training for 20 minutes three times a week is also helpful.

Massage: Can help with lymphatic drainage and detoxification, using a base oil with the addition of essential oils, such as chamomile, rosemary, lavender, ginger, peppermint, and wintergreen. Even Tiger Balm can be useful when applied to the forehead and temples.

Sauna therapy: Detoxing through sweating. Spirochetes do not tolerate heat well. Improved function of the cells helps with oxygen distribution. The increased temperatures also help the body to release endorphins, which are the "feel-good" chemicals in your brain. Endorphins also make great painkillers, so it is very common for people suffering from chronic and acute pain to get quite a bit of relief from sitting in a sauna. The sauna can improve the effectiveness of the immune system as well as kill off many microbes that cannot take the heat; many of them die off at temperatures of 40°C/104°F.

. . . but not so relaxing?

Coffee enemas: In the 1930s a German doctor, Max Gerson, pioneered the use of coffee as part of his healing therapy. He recommended coffee taken rectally, as this can help to dilate the bile ducts and stimulate glutathione in the liver, which helps in removing toxins from the blood stream.

Cold water therapy: Swimming in the sea or cold shower therapy may appear to put your body under stress, but it can, instead, improve vagal tone (see chapter 7) and resilience to stress. It can also reduce inflammation, improve mood, and lift depression. Raising the vagal tone forces the muscles to contract and improves circulation, increasing the blood flow around the body. It takes about three minutes in the water to become comfortable with the cold.

Using herbs alongside conventional treatment

Herbs can be used in conjunction with prescribed treatments, such as antibiotics, to help mitigate the impact of side effects, boost the immune system, and aid recovery after a course of antibiotics. As a herbal practitioner, I am conscious of the interaction between orthodox and herbal treatments.

Managing side effects

Antibiotic treatment can lead to a number of uncomfortable and unpleasant side effects. Using herbs alongside the antibiotics may help to alleviate these, as indicated in Table 4.1.

   Taking probiotics while you are taking antibiotics can be useful to reduce some of the symptoms of bloating and diarrhoea, as well as to repopulate the diminishing beneficial gut bacteria. If clients wish do this, it is best to take them at night, when the digestive tract is resting and healing. Alternatively, eating fermented foods and high-fibre foods on a regular basis as a part of one's diet may be a more cost-effective and beneficial way to replenish the "good" bacteria during antibiotic treatment. This can also establish beneficial eating habits and restore the gut microbiota to a healthy state once the antibiotics course is over.

Table 4.1
Herbs to treat most common side effects of antibiotics

Side effect	Herbal options	Action
Headaches	chamomile, cramp bark, feverfew, Gou Teng, lavender, rosemary, valerian	Massage diluted essence of rosemary or lavender into temples and neck
Headache and visual disturbances	bilberry, cramp bark, ginkgo, Gou Teng	Get eyes checked; wear sun glasses to reduce sensitivity
Mild diarrhoea	chamomile, charcoal, meadowsweet, raspberry	Stay hydrated, avoid caffeine, and stick with bland foods
Feeling or being sick	chamomile or peppermint tea, ginger, Swedish bitters	Drink or eat foods with ginger, little but often; avoid fried food.; bananas or rice may help
Loss of appetite	cinnamon, fennel, ginger, peppermint, prickly ash	Schedule and eat small meals.; bitter herbs help stimulate appetite
Skin sensitive to the sun	aloe vera	Avoid sun; wear protective clothing; use sun screen

Herbs that increase the capacity to recover after taking antibiotics

Health concerns while taking antibiotics can often manifest in some form of imbalance in the billions of microorganism in our body. Candida albicans is a common yeast infection that can result from the use of antibiotics, causing conditions such as thrush; this can occur in the mouth, digestive tract, and vagina. The most common and annoying symptoms include pain, itchy labia, and a white discharge, but signs of thrush can also be seen in white patches on the tongue; sometimes white patches may appear on the skin. Other symptoms include bloating, depression, nasal congestion, and recurrent sore throats. An increase in growth of Candida can also be due to over-use of steroids, a diet high in sugar, carbohydrates, or yeast causing gut dysbiosis, hormonal changes, or long-term use of contraception.

The condition can be made worse by nylon underwear and perfumed body-care products.

Herbal antifungal remedies

Fungal infections are common when taking antibiotics. Infections such as thrush may require both internal and external treatment as they can be difficult to treat; their threadlike network of mycelium can penetrate the gut, causing weakness in cell membranes. Studies have shown that fungal infections are becoming more widespread and aggressive due to over-use of antibiotics.[5] In addition, for those who are immune-compromised, exposure to mould, mycotoxin, and water damage to buildings may also give rise to opportunistic infections, including mould and yeast infections.

Antifungal medicines in tincture form or capsules like olive leaf, calendula, tea tree, oregano, caprylic acid (a coconut-oil extract), Pau d'Arco, garlic, and grape seed extract can keep fungal growth at bay. A herbal plan personalised for an individual will also involve avoiding processed food and including foods that help to re-populate the gut by supporting friendly bacteria in the gastrointestinal tract.

Plants with prebiotic properties include garlic, leek, beetroot, dandelion root, burdock root, marshmallow root, and psyllium seeds. Prebiotics also help to eliminate toxins from the bowel without irritating the lining of the gut. They provide a natural source of soluble fibre and fuel healthy bacteria, thereby strengthening the immune system.

A diet that eliminates food containing yeast, yeast extract, sugar, and carbohydrates, which feed the fungus, may also be helpful.

When fungi or yeast cells are killed off in the body, they release toxins that can make you feel quite ill. Binders are used to help suppress overgrowth and eliminate the endotoxins by binding to toxins that bacteria or fungi can produce, reducing the die-off side effect and preventing reabsorption of toxins in the body. Activated charcoal[6] and Zeolite are popular binders often used to bind to toxins.

There are a number of supplements that can be helpful, such as vitamin C (1–3 g); zinc (15–50 mg a day); high-potency B vitamins (from a non-yeast source); and grape seed extract (5 drops in water a day).

Externally, for thrush, natural yoghurt containing Lactobacillus strains that release hydrogen peroxide, killing the Candida, can be useful. This can be applied to the labia with the fingers, or an unused tampon applicator can be filled with yoghurt and inserted into the vagina, having a cooling effect.

Probiotic pessaries with *Lactobacillus crispatus*, or tea tree and lavender pessaries, can also be applied.

Antifungals: Olive leaf, calendula, Pau d'Arco, garlic.

Essential oils: Tea tree, lavender, oregano.

Herbs to boost the immune system and aid recovery

There are a number of herbs that can help increase the capacity to recover from bacterial infection and become more resilient. The herbs you take and the combinations used will depend on your individual needs. Some people who are sensitive to particular herbs may prefer using single remedies, whereas others like combinations to help reduce symptoms of the illness while boosting the immune system. Some prefer capsules, others liquids.

Most of the herbs are obtained in tincture form from a herbalist or herb supplier. Teas and capsules may be more accessible in shops. Not only are they relatively freely available, they are cheap and effective and have few side effects.

The following herbs can help to boost the immune system and act as herbal antibiotics:

▷ Herbs such as echinacea, elderberry, astragalus, and cat's claw stimulate immune function by increasing white blood cells to control microbial invasion.

▷ Herbs high in nitrates that get converted to nitric oxide can further support immune function by aiding effective cell signalling and activating the immune system in response to a pathogen. This is another efficient way in which plants can have an antibiotic-type effect. Herbs such as turmeric[7] or sweet wormwood (*Artemisia annua*) or oils such as tea tree are effective in this respect. Some plants – for instance, liquorice, horse chestnut, garlic, and red onion – contain saponins (a soap-like substance), which can also break down bacterial or viral cell membranes.

▷ Medicinal plants such as gentian, turmeric, Chelidonium and astragalus inhibit the building blocks that create proteins needed by the bacteria to function.

 ▷ Herbs inhibit the activity of certain enzymes and vitamins, such as folic acid, required for cell division, without which bacteria cannot grow. Green tea and the coniferous tree known as thuja are known to be effective in this way.

 ▷ Some herbs prevent the replication of DNA of bacteria and viruses. Research[8] has shown berberines — chemicals found in plants such as turmeric, goldenseal, Oregon grape (berberis, *Mahonia aquifolium*) — can work in this way.

 ▷ Some herbs inhibit cellular signalling (also known as quorum sensing), stopping the bacterial cells from communicating with each other. This is particularly helpful where there are biofilm formations (communities of bacteria), as these groups of microorganisms can create a type of slimy matrix that behaves like a cloaking device, protecting themselves or the bacteria they cover from being picked up by the immune system. andrographis, garlic, St John's wort, ginger, sweet chestnut, Chelidonium, and ginseng have been shown as inhibiting quorum sensing.

 ▷ Herbs such as liquorice inhibit the binding of the bacteria to cell tissue that can cause disease, impeding *Helicobacter pylori* in attaching to the gut lining,[9] for example. Cranberry inhibits bacteria attaching to the tissue of the bladder.[10] Berberis stops the attachment of bacteria to mucous membranes such as nose, mouth, and gut, and, used topically, to the skin. Berberine has been shown to improve the effectiveness of some antibiotics.[11,12]

 ▷ Some herbs reduce the action of efflux pumps. These pumps might be found in the transport system in a bacteria cell membrane and act to continually remove a drug, such as an antibiotic or herb, from the cell, which means that it never gets the opportunity to fully work. Medicinal plants such as thyme, rosemary,[13] berberis, pomegranate,[14] sweet wormwood (*Artemisia annua*), and Chinese skullcap block and reduce the effect of the pump's regurgitating activity, thus allowing the herb or drug to actually get inside the bacterium and kill it. The use of these plants could increase the bioavailability — the ability of a substance to be absorbed and used by the body — of the targeted drugs or herbs being used to fight the infection.

Natural antibiotics and herbal treatments

There is ever-increasing concern about people becoming resistant to antibiotics and an ever-growing need to use safe and effective alternatives.[15] Health specialists are looking at treatments that can support the immune system to respond to infection without destroying gut health. Encouraging beneficial bacteria to grow can be one way of supporting gut health and the immune system without using antibiotics.

There has been a considerable drop in investment into the research and manufacture of antibiotics over the last two decades. This could be due partly to the decline in government-subsidised projects in antibiotics, which were initiated during the Second World War.[16] Pharmaceutical companies are led by commercial goals, providing incentives to prescribe or finding financial compensation in new discoveries of cures.

On a global level, the increased overuse of antibiotics as medicine for both humans and livestock over the last 60 years has led to antibiotic resistance. Bacteria adapt to survive, thereby lessening the efficacy of the antibiotic.

Beyond antibiotics: supporting the immune response with fungi

Many plants and fungi have effective antibacterial properties that can help improve resistance to infection, and many of the top-selling drugs used in human medicine, including statins and antibiotics, are derived from fungi. Interestingly enough, it may, in fact, be fungi that will help us to cope with antibiotic-resistant bacteria. Scientists at Bristol University have shown mushrooms to be a sustainable source of new antibiotics, because they support our own body. They contain phytonutrients such as beta-glucans, which are polysaccharides: beta-glucans can stimulate the immune system by activating white blood cells, such as macrophages, neutrophils, monocytes, and natural killer cells. Physiologically, they have the ability to improve immune response and antibiotic resistance, to strengthen individual resistance to viral infections, and to improve survival time in some cancer therapies.

Mushrooms have long been esteemed in traditional Chinese medicine for their healing properties. They are all high in both beta-glucans and related polysaccharides and have been useful in improving oxygen supply, supporting the immune response. This is why they are used by oncologists and herbalists in some cancer therapies.

> According to Martin Powell, Chinese herbalist, acupuncturist, expert, and author of numerous books on mushrooms, pre-existing fungal conditions are not a contraindication to eating mushrooms. Indeed, in many cases, consuming mushrooms, either in the diet or as supplements, can have an important role to play in addressing such conditions.

Shiitake mushrooms: Xiang Gu

Shiitake mushrooms were originally grown only in Japan, on natural oak logs. Eaten in stir-fries, soups, and as a meat alternative, they are rich in polysaccharides and lignans and have been used for centuries to prevent collagen deterioration and improve life quality and survival time in cancer treatments. One of their primary roles is to act as an immune modulator and tonic by increasing uptake in nutrients for body weight. (Dose: 1,000 mg [½ tsp]).

Lion's mane (*Hericium erinaceus*)

Lion's mane is a beautiful mushroom. When it grows, it resembles a white waterfall. It has been used by the Chinese to reduce aging effects and menopause-type symptoms such as hot sweats and brain fog and to improve cognitive function.[17] These actions make it particularly helpful for Lyme sufferers, especially to counteract some of the neurological effects of the

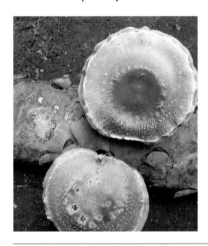

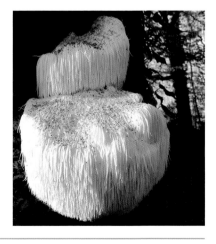

Shiitake   Lion's mane

disease. This mushroom can give some pain relief in diabetic neuropathies or help with that tingling sensation that can cause so much discomfort. This is partially due to compounds that can stimulate the production of nerve growth factor (NGF).

Buhner recommends ½ tsp of the powdered extract three times daily, taken in a small amount of water.

Reishi (*Ganoderma lucidum*)

Reishi, a red, kidney-shaped mushroom, is really helpful in supporting treatment for a wide range of illnesses, and is useful particularly for people with Lyme disease and co-infections, not only because of its adaptogenic properties, helping people combat stress and fatigue, but also because of its antioxidant, antihistamine, anti-inflammatory, antibacterial, and antiviral activity. In various Chinese dynasties, emperors would send their servants out to remote habitats to search for this mushroom because of its reputation of granting them eternal youth and immortality. Reishi was eaten only by royals until cultivation in the twentieth century enabled it to be more accessible to everyone. (Dose: 6–12 g of the raw mushroom per day.)

Turkey tail mushroom (*Trametes versicolor*)

This common and beautiful mushroom looks like a miniature turkey's tail; it is found pretty much everywhere on dead logs. It is used to strengthen the immune system, especially the T helper cells, to detect rogue cells in the body. Turkey tail has helped people with chronic fatigue syndrome, viral meningitis, HIV, HSV, Hep C, and Lyme disease. (Dose: 2 g of the raw mushroom three times daily.)

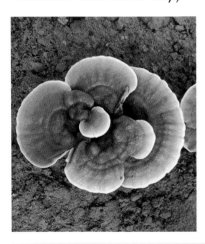

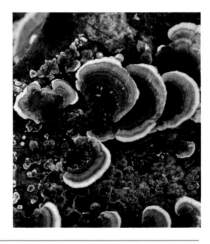

Reishi   **Turkey tail**

Cordyceps (*Ophiocordyceps sinensis*)

Cordyceps has to be one of the strangest mushrooms I have come across. Rather than growing off plants, it grows in an insect host. I first started using it for elderly clients with erectile dysfunction issues or general aches and pains. Later I discovered all of its additional health benefits in supporting people with Lyme disease and recovering from long-term illness, by reducing inflammation with its potent effect of inhibiting NF-κB, which contributes to chronic inflammatory disease.

In China it has been used to regulate sugar levels, heartbeat, and treat viral diseases of the lungs, kidney, and liver. It is used in Lyme disease to restore immune function, support the adrenals, reduce inflammation, and protect mitochondria, due to its ability to improve oxygen supply to the body. It is included as part of the Buhner protocols to increase glutathione levels and reduce oxidative stress in mycoplasma and chlamydia infections.[18] (Dose: 2 g raw mushroom three times daily.)

Herbal treatment

Plants as foods have long been known to have a pharmaceutical effect. The defences of different plants have evolved with the climate and the need of the plant to protect itself. Ironically, it is the constituents of the plant that allow it to protect itself that confer the greatest benefit to us when the plant is eaten. These constituents – known as phytochemicals – are of paramount interest to the medical profession and attract pharmaceutical companies into isolating an active ingredient from a plant and converting it into a drug.

For example, the group of phytochemicals called flavonoids is one of the largest families of polyphenolic compounds; they are further divided into several subclasses. They are often characterised by pigments that give the plants their bright colours. They generally occur in foods such as fruit, vegetables, and herbs, as well as in plant-derived beverages such as tea and wine. Plants produce flavonoids in order to protect themselves against parasites, oxidative injury, and harsh climatic conditions.

It is not surprising that plants can also confer a large range of protections to our bodies, such as antiviral, antibacterial and cardioprotective effects. They can also provide an alternative to corticosteroids and antidepressants and may influence hormone function.

Plants and Lyme disease

This evolutionary kinship between animals, plants, and microbes has been a necessity for survival and healing. The *Borrelia burgdorferi* spirochete is one of the microbes that has been able to adapt to its environment, and this may explain why Lyme disease is so difficult to treat or detect. The corkscrew-like spirochete can change shape into a round body form, also known as a cyst form, and become unrecognised by the immune system. Furthermore, a bacterial film can form around the shape-changed bacterium, protecting it even more from the immune system and detection.

A study published in 2020 in *Frontiers in Medicine* examined the potential of 12 herbs used in treating Lyme disease by testing them *in vitro* for activity against *Borrelia burgdorferi*. The study listed the following 7 plants as the most effective, though I am sure there are many more:

- Ghanaian quinine (*Cryptolepis sanguinolenta*)
- Black walnut (*Juglans nigra*)
- Japanese knotweed (*Fallopia japonica/Polygonum cuspidatum/ Reynoutria japonica*, Hu Zhang)
- Cat's claw (*Uncaria tomentosa*)
- Sweet wormwood (*Artemisia annua*)
- Mediterranean rock rose (*Cistus creticus*)
- Chinese skullcap (*Scutellaria baicalensis*)

This study provides the first convincing evidence that these herbs "have potent activity against Lyme disease bacteria, especially the dormant persister forms, which are not killed by the current Lyme antibiotics".[19]

I first came across these plants in 2005 in Stephen Buhner's book, *Healing Lyme*.[20] I am indebted to his work and recommend this book to all my clients before they come to see me: it is fairly technical and covers the subject in depth. Since 2009, in my practice I have been using many of the plants mentioned in his protocol, with amazing results.

I see a range of clients with Lyme disease. Some have recently been bitten by a tick and have either been identified by their doctor as possibly having Lyme disease, or have themselves been aware of symptoms of bull's-eye rash or flu-like symptoms. They may have received a 2–4-week treatment of antibiotics such as doxycycline. Some clients would like to take herbs to support them while taking antibiotics, to help with side effects, or because they want to be sure they are doing everything they can do holistically to reduce the chance of getting chronic Lyme disease. Many have chosen only to take herbs as a treatment or as a preventative when living in a high-risk area.

Yet for others the disease may not have been diagnosed early enough for antibiotic treatment to be effective. Some I see have been sick for a long time and may have many underlying conditions contributing to their ill health. Often what we, as practitioners, may see are clients who have persistent symptoms being treated by a health care system that feels it has given their patient everything that it can provide at that time.

> "Around 2008, the medical professionals I saw were pretty ignorant of Lyme, and misinformed. When I initially got bitten and ill, my blood tests were negative, no treatment offered. A year later, when I was profoundly ill and the tests confirmed this, I was offered a short course of antibiotics and, strangely, told that I could not have any more. This was before I had had the first course. A short dose cleared up my symptoms nicely, but after a month or two they returned. Further antibiotics had to be forced out of them. They were curious and carried out two lumbar punctures. These were unnecessary for my welfare and made me profoundly ill as for the second they inserted the needle 13 times."

Most clients I see come with a long medical history, large folders, and boxes of supplements. The quote below came from a previously very fit, energetic individual who had been experiencing debilitating symptoms for 11 years, was unable to work regularly, had pages of GP referrals, blood tests, and abnormal blood pressure readings, and was unable to continue medication due to the unbearable side effects.

> "After seven days taking herbal medicine, not a single symptom. I have 100% more energy and haven't felt like this for 11 years; I am more relaxed, happy and smiling – it is a wonderful feeling. I really cannot believe it!

The question as to whether one can treat someone for Lyme disease without using antibiotics is one that often comes up in clinics or on forums. I have used herbs and retested for Lyme disease and results were negative, but that is not uncommon and does not mean the person is suddenly immune to tick bites or Lyme disease. What I can say is that symptoms improve and some go.

The approach of herbal practitioners of treating the whole person and not just the disease has attracted many people to find long-term solutions to improving their health.

"I had been seeing a herbalist and nutritionist for one year or so before being diagnosed with Lyme disease. Bell's palsy, losing sight in one eye, chronic fatigue, shaking and buzzing, sleep deprivation, fibromyalgia, low libido, depression, ringing in ears were just some of the symptoms I was experiencing.

I had my bloods sent to Germany and received a positive Lyme diagnosis. I created a team of a doctor, a nutritionist, and a herbalist. A combination of infusions, herbs, nutraceuticals, diet, and the Lightning Process helped me. I never used antibiotics and believe a combination of treatment helped me get well."

"I have felt physically and emotionally battered during this period of my life, fighting this war with the invisible invaders who always seem to have the upper hand."

As each person is so different, there is no one prescription that fits all. For this reason, when formulating prescriptions, herbalists take the whole person into account and will change their prescription as the symptoms change.

"Long-term herbal treatment was an integral part of my long-term recovery. It took years, but I now enjoy reasonably good health. It has been an incredibly deep hole to dig myself out of, and I have needed and received a huge amount of support.

The absence of habitual and withdrawal symptoms appear more attractive than many of the side effects which may result from taking orthodox drugs."

"I LOVE your sleep mix. Sleep is so essential, really a keystone to all of the other healing, even to having the energy and enthusiasm to make positive change or to believe in yourself."

The plant profiles in chapter 5 provide an easy reference guide to the actions and use of plants and how they can support individuals with Lyme disease.

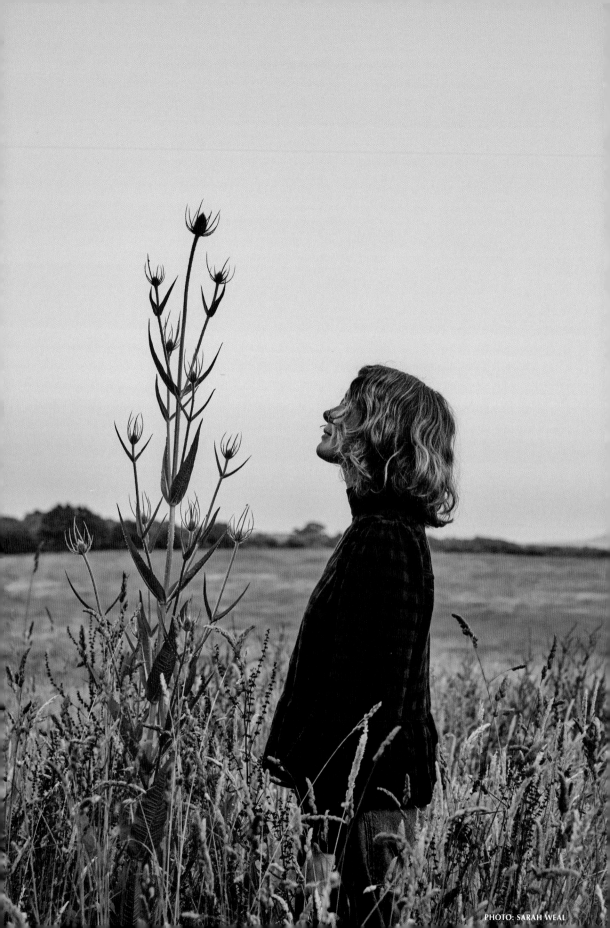

5

Herbal support for Lyme disease: plant profiles

Introduction

For thousands of years before the emergence of laboratory-manufactured pharmaceuticals, medicinal plants had been used as remedies to support and heal. Many of the powerful drugs used in modern medicines originated in plants, and even today many pharmaceutical companies use plant extractions.

Plants are important to pharmaceutical companies both as a source of raw material to incorporate into drugs and as a model for synthetic structure. In the laboratory these companies isolate compounds for use in orthodox medicine, such as morphine from the opium poppy, quinine from cinchona bark, and Taxol from yew tree bark. Herbalists, however, have a different approach when making plant medicine. Their herbal preparations historically use the entire flower, root, leaf, or berry of any plant, with the understanding that there is a synergy between the various plant compounds. It is this balance, coupled with a holistic approach to preparation and treatment, that makes herbal remedies unique.

In contrast to whole-plant preparation, which has been used for centuries, today there appears to be a trend in the herbal industry to make plant preparations resemble pharmaceutical products by isolating the active compounds. These products are then marketed as traditional herbal remedies, which is misleading because traditional herbal remedies contain all the parts of a plant.

The plant profiles in this chapter include all those plants that I use on a regular basis, in combination with many others, when treating clients whose lives have been impacted by Lyme disease.

The profiles present, in a simple form, what plants are like, making them more accessible so you can use them safely to help healing on many different levels. Some of the plants you may recognize growing in your garden, others may be unfamiliar; all can be bought, grown, combined, and administered in a variety of ways.

Preparation

Infusions

Infusions are made from dry or fresh plant material (1 tsp dried = 3 tsp fresh herb). Infusions can be prepared just as you would make a pot of tea: simply by pouring boiling water over a spoonful of herbs – the standard recipe is 30 g dried herb to 500 ml water – and leave to infuse for 5–10 minutes before straining and drinking as specified.

Decoctions

The transformation of the dried form of a herb to a liquid form is called a decoction. Decoctions are usually made using roots, wood, bark, seeds, and/or nuts. The dried material (2–30 g, depending on the plant) is placed in a pan of water and simmered for 15–20 minutes, to make sure all constituents are transferred to the water before straining. The decoction can be kept in a fridge for up to 2 days.

Tinctures

Tinctures are alcohol-based preparations of medicinal plants; they are the most commonly prescribed form of herbal medicine. They keep well and are convenient to take. Alcohol is a better solvent for plant constituents and also acts as a preservative; the percentage of alcohol (e.g., 45% ABV) used will depend on the type of constituents extracted. The quantity of the herb used to the amount of alcohol is usually 1:4 or 1:5 – in other words, for every gram of herb we use 4 or 5 ml of alcohol.

Glycerites

Glycerites are usually used when the client does not want to take, or is sensitive to, alcohol. Dilute the glycerin with distilled water, 3 parts glycerin to 1 part water. Fill two-thirds of a jar with fresh herb/root, or half the jar with dried herb/root. Pour the glycerin + water into the jar to cover the herb and/or root. Leave in a dry, dark place for 6–8 weeks; shake the jar every couple of days. Strain before using use.

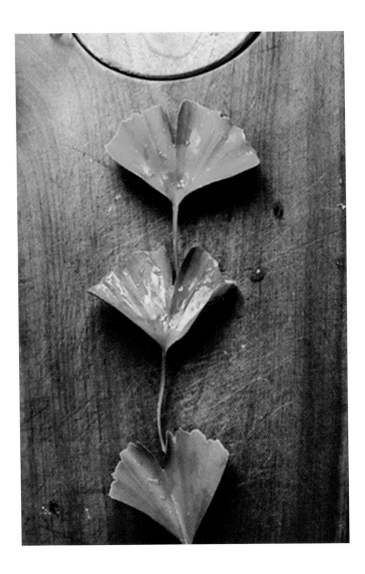

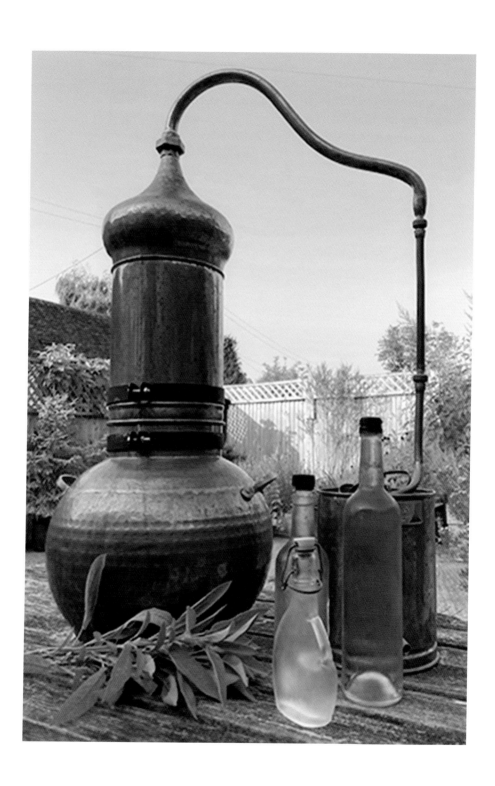

Andrographis * *Andrographis paniculata*

History/traditional use

Andrographis, also known as Chuan Xin Lian, King of Bitters, has been used for centuries for bacterial and viral infections of the respiratory and digestive tract. Some considered it superior to quinine in the treatment of malaria. It has been used for those with weakened immunity, loss of appetite, sluggish digestion or liver, diarrhoea, malaria, and diabetes and to expel toxins from the body.

Action: Antibacterial, antiviral, bitter tonic, cardioprotective, choleretic, hepatoprotective, immunomodulator.

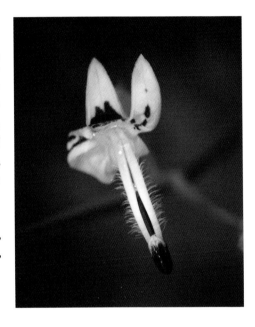

Modern use

Immune system: Andrographis enhances the immune system by stimulating white blood cells, antibodies, and cell-mediated responses to pathogens. Furthermore, research shows that andrographis is able to disrupt the quorum-sensing system (cell-to-cell communication) that bacteria use to latch on to each other and thrive.

Heart: The immune-enhancing function and antioxidant effect of andrographis also has a protective effect on the heart. There is some evidence to suggest that andrographis can reduce high blood pressure and high cholesterol levels. The protective effect to the heart makes it a valuable remedy in Borrelia infections involving the heart and for damage done by the bacteria.

Anti-inflammatory: Andrographis's anti-inflammatory effects and ability to cross the blood–brain barrier, reducing pro-inflammatory proteins, combined with its analgesic effect, can help to reduce swelling and pain.

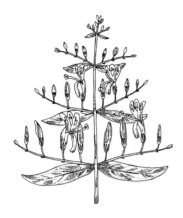

Protective and healing: The hepatoprotective effect on the liver from toxins has been compared favourably to that of milk thistle.

Cultivation

Andrographis is native to India, Sri Lanka, Southeast Asia, China, America, the West Indies, and Christmas Island. It grows well in tropical and subtropical climates and can reach 1 m in height; it prefers fertile, sandy, loam/clay–loam soils and can withstand partial shade.

Harvesting/foraging

Harvest when most of the plant is in flower. The plants can be dried in the sun for two days and afterwards in the shade. The leaf and stem are used to make medicine.

How to use

Decoction: 2–3 g a day, or 6 g a day during infection.

Tincture: 1:3 strength, 2–5 ml, three times a day; or 1:1 strength, 4–6 ml, once a day. Can be taken long-term.

Paste: Make a paste of andrographis tincture mixed with green clay and apply paste to bite; this may help draw out the toxins.

Caution/contraindications

Avoid if pregnant or breastfeeding or if there is a history of stomach ulcers or oesophageal reflux. Generally well tolerated, but can cause urticaria.

Ashwagandha   *   *Withania somnifera*

History/traditional use

In Ayurvedic medicine, ashwagandha has been used to improve and restore balance to the body, improving immune function, fertility, and libido and lifting depression. Its main use is to relieve stress, and it has a balancing and calming effect on the body. It is not surprising that it is called Indian ginseng, because of its rejuvenating effect. It is used by athletes to improve stamina and to increase muscle recovery rate.

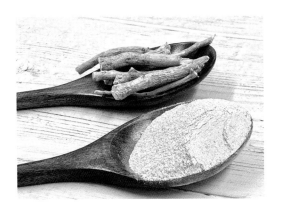

Action: Adaptogenic, anti-anaemic, anticancer, anti-inflammatory, antioxidant, antispasmodic, emmenagogic (stimulating blood flow in the pelvic area), immune-modulating.

Therapists have recommended its therapeutic use in reproductive, respiratory, adrenal, arthritic, and senile disorders.

Modern use

Adrenal support: Helps to regulate stress levels and is commonly used for anxiety and stress.

Its balancing effect can also help to improve cognitive function, stimulate normal thyroid levels, support healthy weight management, and lower blood pressure.

Drug withdrawal: Some studies show that ashwagandha can aid withdrawal from opioid medication due to its sedative effect.[1] I see this, combined with ashwagandha's anti-inflammatory effect, having a huge impact on people suffering with pain and addiction to painkillers that no longer have an effect. "*Somnifera*" means "sleep-inducing" in Latin. It can be used at night, especially when there is stress-induced insomnia or overstimulation.

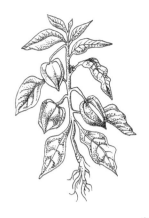

Anti-inflammatory: In Ayurvedic medicine, ashwagandha has a history of being used for lower-back pain, arthritis, skin disorders, and muscle wasting. The tincture has an analgesic and anti-inflammatory effect and does not cause digestive irritation, as some medications do.

Immunity: By stimulating the immune system, ashwagandha has been shown to exhibit anticancer properties and antimicrobial activity against bacteria, fungi, and viruses.

Epstein–Barr virus is often problematic in Lyme sufferers and is often implicated in the causes of chronic fatigue and exhaustion. Studies[2] show that 45% of people suffering from chronic fatigue syndrome showed improvement when taking ashwagandha, as it can enhance physical performance, especially when problems are related to stress. As this plant is also high in iron, it can reduce fatigue and shortness of breath caused by anaemia.

Ashwagandha is used in chemotherapy support and has demonstrated anticancer properties in lung cancer.

Lyme disease: Ashwagandha is often recommended by practitioners where there is nervous exhaustion after stress, chronic illness causing inflammation, or a connective disorder. It is often used in the Buhner protocol for Lyme disease,[3] as it can reduce inflammation while modulating the immune system. Ashwagandha demonstrates inhibitory activity against *Babesia duncani* after three days of incubation *in vitro*.

Ashwagandha has been used to treat the blood-borne pathogens Bartonella and Babesia. As ashwagandha is high in iron, it can help to reduce symptoms of anaemia associated with babesiosis.

When a plant can reduce symptoms of fatigue and improve cognitive function and mood, it goes without saying that it can help to improve multiple symptoms of Lyme disease, its co-infections, and the stressors faced by sufferers.

Cultivation

Grows naturally across India, Asia, and Africa, especially in the drier regions. Prefers sandy well-drained soil; does not like waterlogged soil.

Harvesting/foraging

Roots are ready to harvest after 180 days of growing, when leaves start to dry and berries appear. The root, which has a strong horse-like smell, can be separated to grow on to increase yield of harvest for later use.

How to use

Available as a dietary supplement. Can be added to smoothies. According to Ayurvedic medicine, giving it with warming herbs like ginger or pepper can increase its tonic effect.

Decoction: ½ tsp dried root to 1 litre water; simmer for 10–20 minutes.

Tincture: 1:3 strength (45% ABV), 5 ml, three times a day or at night also effective.

Capsules: >400–500 mg capsules, once or twice per day, or 1–3 tablets half an hour before bed.

Caution/contraindications

Avoid if sensitive to the nightshade family or allergic to nightshade; in that case, you could replace ashwagandha with lemon balm (*Melissa officinalis*). May enhance the effect of benzodiazepine. No contraindication in breast-feeding; in fact, it increases yield. Avoid if suffering from hyperthyroidism.

Astragalus   *   *Astragalus membranaceus*

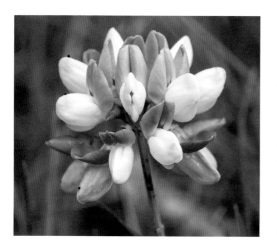

History/traditional use

The root of astragalus – also known as Huang Qi – has been used in Chinese medicine for hundreds of years to prevent infection and for those with impaired immunity. In Chinese and Ayurvedic medicine, it is seen as a strengthening herb that protects most organs in the body. It has traditionally been used to treat bacterial and viral infections, chronic fatigue, high blood pressure, peptic ulcers, congestive heart failure, and nephritis.

Action: Antibacterial, antifungal, antiviral, hypotensive, immune stimulant, rejuvenating tonic for the heart, liver, kidneys, and adrenal glands.

Modern use

Cardiac conditions: Astragalus been used as a cardiac tonic, strengthening the heart and improving conditions such as angina and congestive heart failure. Its potent antioxidant effect suggests that it could be used to improve memory and fatigue and to reduce inflammation.

Immunity: This plant is often used during cancer treatments or after chemotherapy to help support immune function by enhancing natural killer cells that help to destroy cancer cells. There is some evidence to suggest that it can help prolong survival and reduce adverse reactions from some of the toxicity of anticancer drugs.

Astragalus could be taken as a preventative measure during tick season – normally between May and September – by people who work in high-risk areas where deer or ticks are found. The herb is used to boost the person's immune system, preventing the Lyme bacteria from taking a hold in the body in Stages 1 and 2 (see chapter 1). Astragalus can be of benefit in early Lyme disease, but it will make symptoms worse in late Lyme disease. As an antiviral it has been shown to inhibit Coxsackie virus, linked to myocarditis and cardiomyopathy.

Cultivation

A perennial plant, it grows at high altitudes in damp areas and mountainous regions of Korea, Japan, and China. It prefers semi-shady woodlands and cold temperatures.

Harvesting/foraging

The root is dug up and harvested in the autumn of its third year or early spring of the fourth year.

How to use

Often combines well with other herbs, and can be added with other ingredients when making soups.

Lyme disease

Buhner[4] suggests:

Preventative or pre Lyme disease dose:
Capsules: 1,000 mg, two to three times a day, taken if living in high-risk area (equal to 15 ml of tincture).

Active Lyme (Stages 1 and 2):
Capsules: 1,000–4,000 mg, three times a day, for 2–12 months. Tincture: 3–5 ml, 1:5 strength, three times a day.

For new tick bites:
Capsules: Buhner[5] typically recommends taking astragalus 1,000 mg three times a day, increasing to 4,000 mg for 60 days, then reducing. Can be taken for up to 12 months in a high-risk area, if needed.

Paste: The andrographis paste for drawing out toxins from tick bites may be made with astragalus powder in place of green clay.

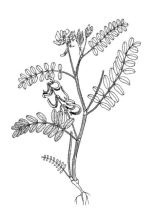

Caution/contraindications

Avoid if taking anticoagulants or immunosuppressant medication.

Avoid in Stage 3 chronic Lyme disease. If Lyme disease is undiagnosed and you have had symptoms for a long while, taking astragalus can make symptoms worse.

History/traditional use

Bidens pilosa has traditionally been used for infections affecting the mucous membranes, whether respiratory or urinary, and conditions such as bronchitis, sore throat, ear and eye problems, stomach pain, rheumatic disease, and muscular pain. In Southern Africa, *Bidens* is used to treat malaria, the symptoms of which are somewhat similar in to Lyme disease. During the Vietnam War, soldiers ate beggar's tick as a vegetable.

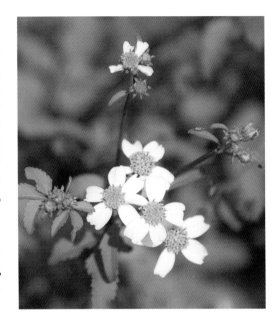

Action: Antibacterial, anticancer, antidiarrhoeal, antifungal, anti-inflammatory, antimalarial, antimicrobial, diuretic, hepatoprotective, hypotensive.

Modern use

More commonly used as an anti-inflammatory and antidiabetic, and to reduce high blood pressure.

Immunity: Beggar's tick is considered an immunomodulator. It helps to protect red blood cells from damage and reduces inflammation and histamine release with allergic asthma and rhinitis.[6]

It also has broad-spectrum antibacterial properties, against both gram-positive and gram-negative bacteria, making it a useful herb when supporting clients with Bartonella, mycoplasma, or penicillin-resistant bacteria.

The diuretic effect of beggar's tick helps the body to flush toxins and eliminate bacteria and thus is useful for the treatment of urinary tract infections and of aching joints similar to gout attacks.

Other active compounds, such as luteolin and linoleic acid, demonstrate antiviral activity *in vitro* and *in vivo;* this is a particularly beneficial herb, inhibiting herpes virus, if there are co-infections with Lyme disease.

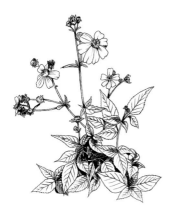

Antifungal properties were found in the root against *Candida albicans*, showing significant potential in treating some of the complications associated with Lyme disease.

Digestion: Beggar's tick has been used around the world in the treatment of diabetes, improving the regulation of insulin production and metabolic syndrome.

Beggar's tick shows significant antimicrobial activity against *E. coli* and *Staphylococcus aureus* and against protozoa microorganisms such as Babesia, and it is useful in gastrointestinal disease.

Skin: Beggar's tick is being developed into skin products, as it is reported as having a retinol-like effect, improving collagen production and protecting the skin against aging and infections.

Cultivation

Fast-growing plant in tropical and warm temperate regions around the world. It is native to Asian countries and the Americas, growing freely along the roadside in coastal areas, along streams, and in agricultural areas.

Harvesting/foraging

Harvest in spring, 3 or 4 times a year, or entire plant, away from roads or from where there are known to be toxins in the ground.

How to use

Leaves are considered a vegetable and can be added to stews; they can be applied externally to wounds or used as a tea or tincture.

Tincture: ½ tsp, three times a day.

Caution/Contraindications

A daily dose of 400 mg, three times a day, for 90 days showed no obvious adverse effects.

Berberis ✳ *Mahonia aquifolium*

History/traditional use

The common name of berberis is Oregon grape. In China, over 3,000 years ago, berberis was used as a bitter herb, in the treatment of gastrointestinal infections affecting the mouth, throat, skin, and gut, especially where there are symptoms of diarrhoea or dysentery. The yellow roots were used both as a medicine and as a dye.

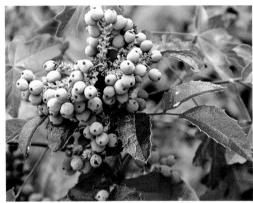

Action: Antidiarrheal, anti-emetic, anti-inflammatory, antimicrobial, antiseptic, astringent, bitter and digestive stimulant, cholagogic (increasing bile secretion), choleretic, hepatic stimulant, hypotensive, immunomodulator, mild laxative, uterine stimulant.

Modern use

The active ingredient in Berberis is berberine, a yellow-coloured, bitter-tasting chemical with strong antibiotic, antifungal, antimicrobial constituents. Berberine is also found in the root and bark of other plants, such as turmeric or goldenseal.

Studies[7] have found berberine to have beneficial effects on the heart and antioxidative activity. Berberine is not easily absorbed with oral administration: you will often find studies that mention injecting berberine.

Immunity: Berberine has been seen as an immune modulator rather than stimulator: it reduces over-activity of the immune system. Berberine-containing plants interfere with gram-positive and gram-negative bacteria attaching onto mucous membranes and replication of certain types of bacteria, fungus, and viruses. Studies have shown berberine to be effective in 20 strains of *Candida* spp.[8] Other studies report benefit to reduce strains of certain type of acne, *E. coli*, staphylococci,[9] and MRSA[10] infection.[11]

Synergy with drugs and herbs: Berberis could be seen as a novel tool working synergistically with fluconazole (antifungal), ampicillin (antibiotic used for treating MRSA), or oxacillin (a penicillin antibiotic),[12] as it improves the effectiveness of the antibiotic.[13] This can contribute to inhibiting the effect of the efflux pump, which keeps pumping drugs out of the bacteria cell and affects the permeability of the cell membrane. Sweet wormwood can enhance this effect.[14]

Berberine becomes more absorbable when combined with liquorice, and thus more effective in the body. This, combined with liquorice's antiviral and anti-inflammatory action and affinity to the gut, can make this combination particularly useful in many viral conditions.

Sweet wormwood (*Artemisia annua*) can also work synergistically to increase the effectiveness of berberine, as well as having the effect of destabilising the cell membrane of the bacteria giving the antibiotic more of a chance to get into the cell and kill the bacteria. Berberine can also inhibit DNA replication of certain bacteria and reduce the growth of bacteria.

Blood sugar: Numerous studies have shown a reduction in blood sugar with berberine: inhibiting absorption of sugars from the intestine and enhancing production of insulin and reducing damage to cells, as well as reducing fasting glucose and cholesterol levels.[15] Not only does the improved insulin sensitivity inhibit fat storage, berberine also improves gut flora, which is a key factor in preventing obesity.[16] A human study with patients taking 500 mg of berberine three times a day for 12 weeks showed a drop in weight of 2.25 kg and in cholesterol levels.[17]

This can be really helpful in conditions such as diabetes, obesity, and polycystic ovaries (PCO).[18] The therapeutic effect of berberine over three months can have a blood lipid lowering effect and can support people with metabolic disorders and improve insulin resistance.[19]

Anti-inflammatory: Berberine studies[20] with chronic hepatitis sufferers have also shown reduction in inflammatory markers and liver damage. Berberis extracts have been used topically for chronic inflammatory skin disease such as acne and psoriasis, reducing the proliferation of lesions.

Cultivation

There are over 70 Berberis species throughout the world. Berberis has a yellow woody stem and dark green, glossy, spiky alternate leaves 25 cm long (looks a little like holly). The flowers are yellow, 5–10 cm, with blue-black berries.

Harvesting/foraging

Fruits in late spring. If harvesting berries, be careful to avoid the spikes. Harvest the root in late winter, after seeds have appeared. Young plants can be pulled up by holding the base of the stem; older roots will need to be dug out with a fork.

How to use

Using 25% alcohol for extraction is suitable for certain conditions, but a high alcohol content (70%) is needed to extract berberine from the plant.

Powder: 3–6 g of dried root a day may be used for topical application or as a douche or wash.

Tincture: 1:1 strength, 3–6 ml a day; 1:2 strength, 3½–7 ml a day.[21]

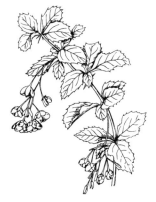

Caution/contraindications

Berberis is contraindicated in pregnancy and lactation. It interacts with immunosuppressive drugs such as cyclosporine and is contraindicated for those with obstructed bile ducts. The berberine effect on drugs can also inhibit the action of monoamine oxidase – a drug often used for depression.

Black walnut ✳ *Juglans nigra*

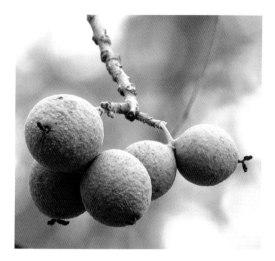

History/traditional use

Black walnut is native to North America; it was introduced to Europe in 1629. Some may be familiar with this large tree, as one of its primary uses has been in the making of cabinets and furniture. Native Americans used the husks as a treatment against parasites and mosquitoes, and for bacterial infections such as diphtheria and syphilis. The black walnut is considered more potent than the English walnut.

Action: Antifungal, antioxidant, antiparasitic, antitumour, chemoprotective.

Modern use

Heart: Common walnuts are high in vitamin E and have been used to improve cardiac health and diabetes, to reduce cholesterol, and to rid the body of infections. The black walnut contains arginine, which can turn into nitric acid; this has a vasodilation effect, which may have a potential for lowering blood pressure.

Brain: The brain shape of the walnut has always alluded to its use inside the body, and science has found antioxidant properties and polyphenols that have shown anti-inflammatory effects on the brain, potentially having a positive impact on neurodegenerative diseases.

Gut health: Black walnut aids digestion, protects the liver, and improves bile flow. It is nutritionally high in folic acid, vitamin B5, vitamin B6, and omega-3 fatty acids. Its antibacterial properties are effective against *Staphylococcus aureus*. It reduces intestinal parasites and helps in expelling worms such as ringworm, pinworm, and tapeworm from the intestines.

There is some evidence to suggest that it can aid in the suppression of colon cancer.

Lyme disease: Black walnut is being used in Lyme therapy for its anti-spirochete and antiparasitic effect; there is also some evidence suggesting that it is effective against biofilms and other co-infections, including viruses.

An immune modulatory effect combined with the broad anti-inflammatory properties may provide some relief in symptoms to some people suffering from long-term Lyme disease.

Black walnut's laxative effect means it is often used in a cleanse, expelling intestinal parasites.

People with Lyme disease have often had a history of antibiotic use and are susceptible to yeast overgrowth. The antifungal properties of black walnut can assist with reducing the side effects of taking antibiotics.

Harvesting/foraging

Unripe walnut husks are peeled from around the fruit (this can stain your hands). They are used for their anti-inflammatory and antiparasitic activity, whereas the inner bark has a more laxative and emetic effect. The walnut husks are hulled mechanically and hung up to dry at 24°C for 15 days, then powdered. The kernels removed from the shell can be ground in a coffee grinder.

How to use

Black walnut can be used as a gargle; it can also be painted on wounds to reduce infections.

Tincture: 1:3 strength (45% ABV), 10–60 drops, three times a day; or 500 mg, three times a day, for 30 days. Take 2 hours before or after medication or supplements.

Nasal rinse for mould spores: 20 drops black walnut tincture in a cup of water; rinse nasal passages two to three times a day.

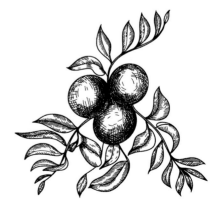

Caution/contraindications

Side effects are usually well tolerated. Can have a laxative effect. Long-term doses have a purging effect, so normally consider only for the short term. Avoid if allergic to nuts, or if pregnant.

Cat's claw ✳ *Uncaria tomentosa*
Gou Teng ✳ *Uncaria rhynchophylla*

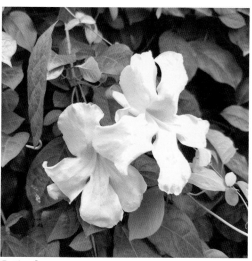
Cat's claw

History/traditional use

Traditionally, cat's claw was used as a tonic in the treatment of weakness and fatigue, asthma, urinary tract infections, kidney disorders, digestive disorders, gastric ulcers, cancer, shingles, skin disorders, cirrhosis, high blood pressure, arthritis, and muscle pain.

Action:

Cat's claw (*Uncaria tomentosa*): Analgesic, antibacterial, anticoagulant, antidepressant, anti-inflammatory, antineoplastic, antioxidant, antiviral, cholesterol-lowering, diuretic, immunomodulator (lowering activated immune response where necessary, as well as enhancing immune function), wound healing.

Gou Teng (*Uncaria rhynchophylla*): antibacterial, anticonvulsant, anti-inflammatory, antiviral, hypotensive, neurologically protective, relaxant, sedative.

Modern use

More recently, cat's claw and Gou Teng have been used during the treatment of Lyme disease, arthritis, and immune deficiencies.

Cat's claw and Gou Teng contain some of the same alkaloids, albeit in different quantities, the latter having a greater ability to reduce neurological symptoms such as dizziness, vertigo, tremors, fevers, seizures, high blood pressure, and headaches.

Lyme disease: There is some evidence to suggest cat's claw raises the white blood cell count and CD57 and natural killer cells. Low CD57 levels are diagnostic markers for some chronic conditions, including Lyme disease.

Lee Cowden and colleagues[22] conducted a pilot study in 2003 with Lyme clients taking cat's claw. This showed an 85% reduction in Lyme disease when patients were retested after six months. Some considered the study flawed as patients had taken antibiotic treatment in the past and as a variety of methods were used in healing at the time, not just cat's claw.

Anti-inflammatory: Research indicates use in reducing inflammation in the digestive system and joint tissue. A clinical trial over 4 weeks with 45 participants suffering from knee pain showed significant improvement: 15 people tested were given a placebo, and 30 people tested were given cats claw. Pain scores and inflammatory markers were reduced after first week of treatment for those who took cat's claw.[23]

Cardiovascular tonic: Due to its vasodilating properties, it can lower blood pressure, reduce clotting, and lower heart rate and cholesterol levels.

Cultivation

Cat's claw is a tropical woody vine that grows in South American forests. Gou Teng, in the same family but a different species, grows in Japan and in China.

These species are typical of tropical and subtropical humid climates, needing favourable weather conditions and temperatures of 17.0–25.7°C in a moist, wet atmosphere. The seeds have a very short viability but can be grown in Europe in greenhouses.

Harvesting/foraging

The inner bark of the vine is harvested. There is severe overharvesting of this herb including digging up the root, even though it is the inner bark that is primarily used in medicine.

How to use

Tincture: 1:5 strength (60% ABV); or administered as a decoction. As little as 1–10 drops may be needed, depending on personal response.

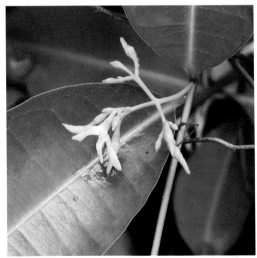

Gou Teng

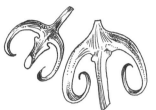

> ▷   Cat's claw: 0.5–5 ml, three to six times a day, for its arthritic properties and to reduce inflammation.
> ▷   Gou Teng: 1:5 strength (60% ABV), 0.5–5 ml, three to six times a day; can be increased if neurological symptoms are present; should be reduced with low blood pressure.

Decoction: Traditional dosage is a decoction of 10–15 g, three times a day.

Capsules: 3–4 500-mg capsules, three to four times a day, maintained for 18 months.

Caution/contraindications

Digestive complaints such as loose stools: reduce dose or discontinue if symptoms persist. Do not use if you are pregnant or about to undergo surgery, taking blood thinners or taking immunosuppressant drugs, or have low blood pressure.

The PAO controversy with cat's claw refers to a debate over standardising cat's claw supplements to contain a specific percentage of pentacyclic oxindole alkaloids (PAOs), a group of compounds found in cat's claw that are believed to be responsible for its medicinal properties. Some argue that PAO standardisation ensures consistency and potency, while others argue that it ignores other bioactive compounds in cat's claw. There is also debate over the best method for measuring PAO content in cat's claw supplements. As a result, consumers should be cautious when purchasing cat's claw supplements and consult with a healthcare professional before using them.

Chinese skullcap * *Scutellaria baicalensis*

History/traditional use

Chinese skullcap (*Scutellaria baicalensis* — not to be confused with *Scutellaria lateriflora*) has been used in traditional Chinese medicine for over 1,500 years to treat diarrhoea, insomnia, inflammation, hypertension and respiratory infections.

Action: Anti-anxiety, antibacterial, anticancer, anticonvulsant, antidiarrhoeal, antifungal, antihistamine, anti-inflammatory, antioxidant, antispasmodic, antitumour, antiviral, astringent, expectorant, haemostatic, hepatoprotective, immune modulator, nervine, neuroprotector, sedative.

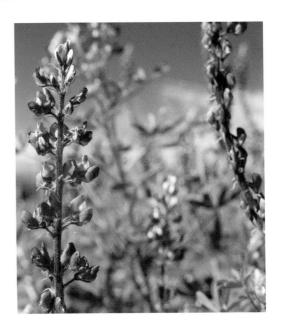

Modern use

Lyme disease: Chinese skullcap can enhance the activity of herbs and drug absorption. This is particularly beneficial during antibiotic use.

Enhance immunity and protection: Benefits include improved immune detection, cell regulation, DNA repair, reducing allergic reactions and inflammatory cascades while protecting nerve tissue and the liver.

Important are its antiviral and antifungal effects, making it particularly beneficial for those who are suffering from herpes viruses or Candida.

The root has also shown promise in treating co-infections such as mycoplasma, Bartonella, and chlamydia infection.

Used as a preventative medicine for respiratory infections, allergies such as rhinitis, hay fever, inflammatory skin conditions. Also indicated for its anti-inflammatory effect, particularly when it comes to autoimmune and digestive disorders or infections of the gut or urinary system.

Increase absorptions: Increases absorption of vitamin C, vitamin E, and glutathione, protecting and repairing tissue, especially in the brain.

Cultivation

Native to China, it can also be found in Russia, Japan, Korea, and Mongolia. Loves sunny to part-shady conditions, and light, well-drained (but not dry) soil. Can be grown from seed straight outside, or inside before it is ready to be transplanted outdoors. Chinese skullcap is not a fussy plant, although it thrives in cooler climates.

Harvesting/foraging

The roots may be harvested from 3–4-year-old plants in spring and autumn. You may wish to dry the roots in a fairly dry, partly shaded, and well-ventilated area.

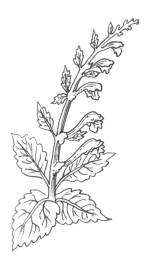

How to use

Decoction: 3–9 g daily.

Capsule: 400–1,000 mg, two or three times a day; or 5:1 concentrated capsules, one to three times a day, depending on the condition.

Tincture: An alcohol concentration of 70% ABV is best.

Caution/contraindications

Avoid with anticoagulants, CNS depressants, or hypoglycaemic medication, or during first trimester of pregnancy.[24]

History/traditional use

The Spanish Jesuit missionaries exploring Peru during the 1600s were introduced to the use of cinchona tree bark to treat malaria and suppress parasites. Cinchona is also known as Jesuit bark or Peruvian bark. Various *Cinchona* species are used, including *C. officinalis* and *C. calisaya*.

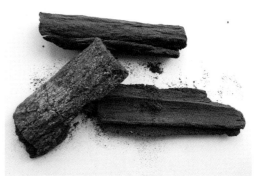

Action: Anti-arrhythmic, antibacterial, anti-fungal, anti-inflammatory, antimalarial, antipyretic, antiviral.

Modern use

Malaria and Lyme disease: In the 1820s, quinine – the medication used to treat malaria and babesiosis – was isolated from the cinchona bark. Babesia, a co-infection of Lyme disease, is a genus of parasitic protozoa that infect red blood cells and cause a disease called babesiosis, which can be transmitted to humans by tick bites. While babesiosis and malaria share some similarities, they are caused by different types of parasites and have different transmission routes. Cinchona has, however, been used to reduce the malaria-like symptoms of Babesia pathogens.

Aching joints: The origins of hydroxychloroquine, a drug being used for malaria and arthritis, originated from the cinchona bark. It helps regulate the activity of the immune system, reducing inflammation pathways, joint swelling, stiffness, and parasites.[25] It has been used for decades to treat Lyme disease, nocturnal leg cramps, rheumatoid arthritis, lupus, and juvenile arthritis. It is thought that one way it inhibits joint pain is by slowing the response to the chief neurotransmitter, acetylcholine, which causes muscle contractions.[26]

Heart: As cinchona can block the sodium channels, it can reduce heart arrhythmias. This works best when there is an onset of arrhythmia, and it can lower blood-pressure levels. This is dose-dependent, and the toxic dose is close to the active dose, so *it can only be used under medical supervision.*[27]

Antiviral: Quinine has antiviral activity against herpes simplex, influenza A, and Dengue fever. Cinchona bark, when combined with zinc, has the potential of stopping viral replication.

Cultivation

Cinchona is a perennial. It grows in open woodland, often in forests where there is cloud cover, and reaches 90–120 cm in height in fertile, well-drained soil.

In South America, native to the mountains in the southern portion of the Andes. Also found in plantations in Africa, Tanzania, Cameroon, Congo, and Rwanda.

Harvesting/foraging

Harvest the dark reddish brown flat quills, about 30 cm long, 1–4 cm wide, 3–4 mm thick. They have a particular odour.

How to use

This bitter-tasting bark is used in tonic water – a popular mixer with gin – containing a 0.03% low dose of quinine, flavouring the water.

This is a restricted Schedule 20 Part 2 herb as defined in the Human Medicines Regulations 2012.[28] It can be prescribed only by a qualified medical herbal herbalist, medical doctor, or pharmacist. According to most practitioners, it is not recommended for more than 1 month because of its potent cardiac toxicity, which can be fatal.

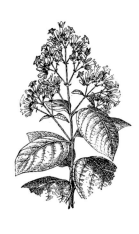

Capsules: 250 mg (Maximum single dose, MD); 750 mg (Maximum daily dose)

Tincture: The maximum dose of a 1:10 strength (45% ABV), is 50 ml per week; maximum daily dose is 7 ml a day, so a dose of 1 ml, three times a day, is a safe starting dose.

Can be taken over a period of 7 days when symptoms are worse, but for a much shorter time by hypersensitive people.

Caution/Contraindications

Side effects include nausea, vomiting, tinnitus, vasodilation, sweating, headache, arrhythmias, and impairment of cranial nerve VIII, leading to symptoms such as vertigo, visual disturbances, decreased auditory acuity, bilateral vision loss. Can have an effect on blood platelets in some people. Contraindicated for those with clotting disorders, cardiac problems, maculopathies, myasthenia gravis, erythema multiform; it may lower blood sugar levels by stimulating insulin secretion, so caution is needed if diabetic.

According to Afifah Hamilton,[29] a single 1.5–2 g dose can be fatal.

Cinnamon   ✳   *Cinnamomum zeylanicum*

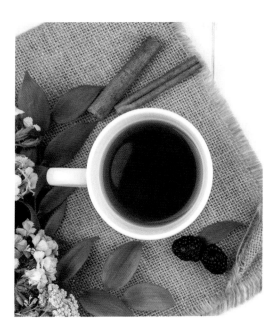

Historical/traditional use

Cinnamon is an aromatic evergreen tree with oval-shaped leaves. Another type of cinnamon is cassia (*Cinnamomum aromaticum*). The two are similar in use.

The bark of the cinnamon tree (*Cinnamomum zeylanicum*) has been used as a medicine and food. Its sweet and spicy flavour was also used by the wealthy in ancient Egypt to embalm and protect mummies. In traditional medicine cinnamon was used for its calming effect on the digestive system, easing bloating, diarrhoea, and nausea and soothing toothaches; also used to stop heavy bleeding during birth or flooding during a period or miscarriage.

Action: Antidiabetic, anti-inflammatory, antimicrobial, antioxidant, antiseptic, astringent, carminative, cholesterol lowering.

Modern use

Lyme disease: Cinnamon's traditional use of boosting the immune system and regulating blood sugar levels could have significant benefits in supporting people with Lyme disease, including reducing brain fog.

Boosting the immune system: Cinnamon's antimicrobial properties not only protect the tree itself from pests and disease; the essential oils found in it have proved to be effective against fungi and multi-drug resistant bacteria.

Improving sugar control: Cinnamon has been linked to reducing the risk factors associated with Type 2 diabetes. It does this by lowering the amount of glucose entering the blood stream, increasing insulin sensitivity, lowering cholesterol, enhancing its antioxidant effect, and reducing inflammation.

Gut health: The antibacterial effect can also inhibit bacterial overgrowth, and it has been seen as having a prebiotic effect in the gut.

Oral health: Cinnamon was one of the original antimicrobial toothpastes used to prevent tooth decay.

Brain health: Compounds in cinnamon appear to be beneficial not only in protecting the neurons in the brain, but also in reducing the build-up in the brain of Tau, a protein that contributes to Alzheimer's disease. This may lead to other therapeutic discoveries and approaches in using this spice with Parkinson's and Alzheimer's disease.

Cultivation

Cinnamon grows in the tropics and is native to Sri Lanka, Vietnam, Bangladesh, and Burma, with large cultivation in and export from China.

Harvesting/foraging

The bark can be harvested from 1–3-year-old branches. When dried, it naturally curls into quills. The smaller stems can have the outer bark scraped off and also be used.

How to use

Tea: 1 tsp dried cinnamon to one cup of boiling water to make a tasty tea. Infuse for 5–10 minutes.

Tincture: 1–3 ml, up to three times a day, in a little water, unless told otherwise by a qualified herbal medicine practitioner.

Capsules: 2 g per day may be taken as a powder or capsules.

Cinnamon toothpaste:

2 tsp arrowroot

1 tsp cinnamon powder

- Mix the ingredients together; be sure to label the container.
- If you prefer to use paste rather than powder, add the above ingredients and just sufficient witch hazel to produce a stiff paste.

Caution/Contraindications

Rare. Avoid if allergic to it. Also avoid large doses during pregnancy as it may have an emmenagogue effect. Because cinnamon lowers blood sugar levels, these should be monitored if taking hypoglycaemic medication.

Garlic * *Allium sativum*

History/traditional use

The origins of garlic are in Central Asia, but it is now cultivated all over the world and is a natural part of people's diet worldwide. In Ancient Egypt, it was given to slaves to give them the strength to build pyramids. In the Second World War it was used to ease dysentery and ward off colds. It has been used for decades to strengthen the heart. The properties of wild garlic (*Allium ursinum*) are similar to those of regular garlic.

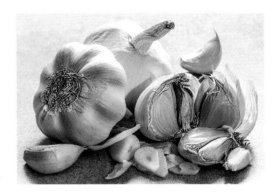

Action: Antibacterial, antifungal, anti-inflammatory, antiseptic, anti-spirochete, diaphoretic, diuretic, expectorant, heavy metal chelator.

Modern use

Garlic is used for its broad-spectrum antimicrobial activity and for being protective against heart disease and cancer.

Detoxification: Raw garlic can stimulate the liver and digestion. It is protective of oxidative damage to red and white blood cells, particularly if there is metal toxicity. It is one of the top plants to increase detoxification levels and raise glutathione, which supports liver detoxification pathways and the removal of toxins and pathogens from the body.

Immune system: Garlic can be used for the treatment of infections. By drying secretions and removing toxins, it tends to give relief from colds, catarrh, rhinitis, intestinal and fungal infections, eruptions, and boils.

It can inhibit bacterial infections and help reduce communication (quorum sensing) between bacteria, including in biofilms.

The antifungal effect of garlic may be of interest to those on antibiotics, especially where these have to be taken for long periods.

Garlic oil has been shown in studies[30] to have antibacterial properties against Lyme disease.

Antiviral against influenza B and herpes simplex, but not against Coxsackie viruses.

Garlic's wide-ranging effect on enzymes also reduces inflammation in the body.

Heart health: Garlic is one of the cheapest and most easily accessible plants to support cardiovascular health. Even though a rare occurrence, Bartonella and Borrelia bacteria can affect the heart; a cardiovascular tonic like garlic could be protective and restorative. Garlic is an antioxidant that can reduce oxidative stress on the body. It acts as an anti-clotting agent, decreases LDL cholesterol, and lowers blood pressure.

Cultivation

Prefers rich, well-drained, sandy soil. Plant a clove in the soil when the ground is cold in early spring, autumn, or winter.

Harvesting/foraging

Gather when the leaves start to turn brown and die down. You can harvest between May and October, depending on when you had sown.

How to use

Can have a powerful antibiotic effect if taken on an empty stomach or with other herbs.

Preventative dose: Take one crushed clove of raw garlic on rising every day. Higher doses (2–5 g) are recommended for infection.
A clove two or three times a day for six days with some oregano oil is sometimes used as part of a seed-and-weed protocol that encourages healthy bacteria back into the gut.

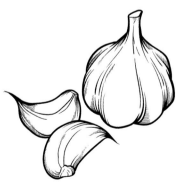

Capsules: 1–3 capsules of freeze-dried powder.

Tincture: 3 ml (60 drops), three times a day.

Caution/Contraindications

There is no evidence of incompatibilities with other medication, but the potential anticoagulant effect is worth noting or allergies related to the sulphur compounds.

Ghanaian quinine * *Cryptolepis sanguinolenta*

History/traditional use

Traditionally, the plant was used in central and western Africa to manage various forms of malaria, fevers, jaundice, hepatitis, digestive disorders, and some amoebiasis, as well as infections caused by bacteria, and to relieve stomach complaints, amoebic dysentery, and diarrhoea. In Ghana, it is grown specifically to support people who suffer from malaria.

Action: Antibacterial, antidiabetic, antifungal, anti-inflammatory, antiprotozoal, antithrombotic, antiviral, vasodilatory effects.

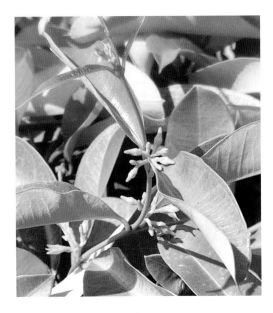

Modern use

Lyme disease: Ghanaian quinine demonstrates a wide range of antimicrobial activity, making it a popular herb in the Americas against Borrelia and opportunist infections associated with Lyme disease, such as Babesia, viruses, and fungi.

Preclinical studies[31] *in vitro* have shown a 7-day treatment with 1% Ghanaian quinine could eradicate *B. burgdorferi* bacterium.[32] This antimicrobial plant is often compared to the antibiotic cefuroxime.

Ghanaian quinine has been used to treat a number of inflammatory conditions, including arthritis. It can therefore help with the following aspects of Lyme disease: fever, respiratory or stomach complaints, malaria-type symptoms, and inflammation of the brain and joints similar to the inflammation you find with arthritis and rheumatism.

Bark of the root or root extracts shows larger antimicrobial and anti-inflammatory properties than the leaf, which is used as an antifungal agent.

Malaria: Ghanaian quinine was one of the first antimalarial drugs made. The antimalarial properties of quinine were discovered in the cinchona tree.

Ghanaian quinine is used against chloroquine-resistant *Plasmodium falciparum* strains. Malaria and Lyme disease are both caused by spirochetes.

Some symptoms of malaria, such as the fevers, chills, aches, and pains, are very similar to those of Lyme disease, so it is not surprising the two diseases have similar treatments.

Regulating sugar levels: Cryptolepine, a chemical compound found in the root, has been shown to reduce fasting blood glucose and body weight and to support regeneration of pancreatic cells.

This demonstrates the plants potential in regulating blood sugar levels in Type 2 diabetes. This also suggests it can further support Lyme clients with regulating blood glucose.

Cultivation

Ghanaian quinine grows largely in tropical rainforests on the western coast of Africa, where there is enough rainfall. It is difficult to grow unless seeds are fresh and there is enough rainfall.

Harvesting/foraging

Because of forest clearing and non-sustainable harvesting, this root should be obtained from a sustainable source and not harvested from the wild.

The yellow root varies from 0.4 to 6.6 cm in length and from 0.31 to 1.4 cm in width and has a sweet fragrance.

How to use

Higher concentrations of alcohol (90% and 60% ABV ethanol extracts) have better inhibitory effect.

Roots and leaves are chewed.

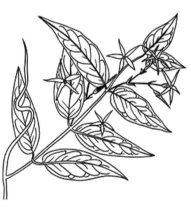

Tincture: 1:2 strength, 10–20 drops, four times a day maximum (1:5 strength, 65% ABV) or 5 ml, three times a day, for 60 days.

Ghanaian quinine is considered to have the effect of an antibiotic for some people, and they may respond very strongly to it, so it is important to adjust, lowering the dose accordingly and making it easier to take.

Caution/contraindications

Avoid during pregnancy. Avoid if wanting to conceive, as it may lower testosterone levels. It may have a purging effect.

Ginkgo * *Ginkgo biloba*

History/traditional use

Geological records show us that ginkgo has been growing on the earth for 150–200 million years, making it one of the oldest living species in the plant kingdom. Chinese monks have cultivated ginkgo since ancient times and have held it sacred in their Buddhist temples. This has presumably ensured the survival of this species.

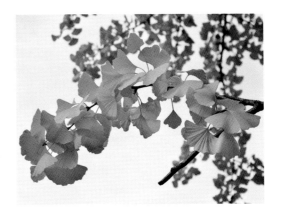

Action: *Leaves:* circulatory stimulant, vasodilator; *seeds;* antibacterial, antifungal, astringent.

Modern use

Lyme disease: Ginkgo is one of the top-ten over-the-counter sellers in the United Kingdom, United States, and Germany for memory loss and cognitive function, both of which can also be aspects of Lyme disease.

Cardiovascular system: Ginkgo is most commonly used to improve blood flow. It does this by affecting the flow of calcium, stimulating the relaxation and contractibility of muscle tissue on the blood vessel of the artery wall. This can reduce the effect of long-term damage caused by reduced oxygen supply to the muscle tissue. There are many studies[33] to suggest that ginkgo may improve outcomes for patients with acute ischemic strokes.

Ginkgolides block platelet activating factor, which would otherwise increase inflammation and the stickiness of red blood cells. The flavonoids are anticoagulant, dilate blood vessels, inhibit lipoxygenase, and reduce inflammation.

Ginkgo regulates sugar and energy levels in the brain, especially in those deprived of oxygen.

Its antioxidant effect of mopping up free radicals can reduce damage to cells and protect organs.

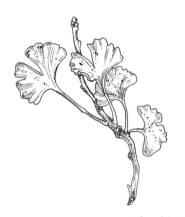

Alzheimer's disease: Ginkgo is gaining recognition for improving memory loss, vertigo, tinnitus, and fatigue, and it has been particularity useful in the treatment of Alzheimer's disease, helping to improve cognitive function.

The German Commission E has approved the extract to be used to treat dementia and symptoms of impaired memory. Needs to be used for 4–6 weeks before benefits are seen.

Tinnitus: Ginkgo has been seen to give moderate improvement to symptoms of tinnitus, which can have considerable benefits to a person's quality of life. Standardised ginkgo extract was shown to have a superior effect when compared to placebo.[34]

Cultivation

Ginkgo is generally grown as an ornamental tree, reaching over 7 m in height. The female trees are less popular, as there is often an unpleasant smell from the fallen fruit. The trees are suitable for coastal areas and are also grown as street trees, in countries such as the United States, Canada, and Australia and in many European countries. They are known for their ability to tolerate a wide range of environmental conditions, including air pollution, making them a popular choice for urban landscapes.

Harvesting/foraging

The leaves are harvested in midsummer, before they change colour.

How to use

Tea: 4–16 g leaf a day, infuse for 5–10 minutes.

Tincture: 1:3 strength, 3–6 ml a day.

Caution/contraindications

Gingko should not be taken if you are already using blood thinners. Stop taking two weeks before surgery.

Hawthorn * *Crataegus monogyna*

History/traditional use

In Britain hawthorn was referred to as fairy apples, or the bread-and-cheese tree: the berries were eaten in times of hardship. The ancient Greeks used hawthorn for heart problems. A closely related species is the Midland hawthorn, *Crataegus laevigata*,

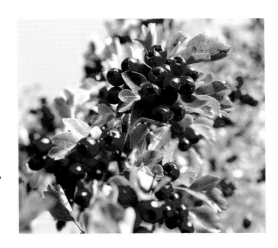

Action: Antioxidant, cardiac tonic, coronary vasodilator, hypotensive.

Modern use

In Europe, thousands of doctors prescribe hawthorn for the prevention of cardiovascular disease. Today, hawthorn is mainly used as a tonic to treat angina, hypertension, atherosclerosis, and arrhythmias and may support people with insomnia or nervous conditions, or as a preventative medicine for those with a family history of cardiovascular problems.

Cardiac health: Hawthorn leaf, flowers, and berries are often combined and have been used for feelings of tightness or pressure from the heart, palpitations raising heart-beat, and vertigo.

Blood pressure: Hawthorn contains a compound when taken internally that stimulates nitric oxide to be released. The release of nitric oxide from the thin cell membranes that line the blood vessels is important for cell signalling and blood vessel health. This has a dilating effect on blood vessels, which, in turn, can lower blood pressure. Low nitric oxide in the body is associated with heart disease, high blood pressure, and diabetes.

Antioxidant: Hawthorn is high in flavonoids and antioxidants, which help reduce the risk of heart disease. The antioxidant effect protects heart tissue against shortage of oxygen and strengthens the blood vessels, stimulating cross-linking of collagen and dilating blood vessels.

Clinical trials: A clinical trial compared a medication called Capto-pril, which lowers blood pressure, to hawthorn extract. One group took

900 mg of Captopril a day for two months, while the other group took hawthorn extract; the results were similar in lowering blood pressure, but the hawthorn group had fewer side effects.

Cultivation

The common hawthorn is a shrubby tree in the rose and apple family, with both long and short roots; the short roots are thorny. The plant has small white-to-pink flowers. It is very commonly found as a hedge plant throughout Britain, North America, Europe, and Asia, supporting over 300 insects.

Harvesting/foraging

Gather flowers and leaf in May, berries in autumn.

   The flowers, with or without leaves, should be dried quickly but gently. The berries require drying slowly with little heat. Both are then best used as a tea, though the fruit will need to be boiled a little first.

How to use

Tea: 30 g per litre water, 1–3 teacups, taken three times per day.

Tincture: 1:5 strength, 3–15 ml a day.

No adverse effects are expected; minimum use 6 weeks to see results.

Caution/contraindications

The German Commission E – a governmental regulatory agency that consists of scientists, toxicologists, physicians, and pharmacists – approved

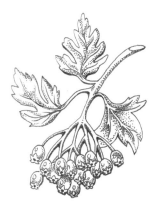

hawthorn products made from the leaves and flowers as effective for patients with reduced cardiac performance. However, if on medication such as hypoglycaemic or hypotensive drugs, the use of hawthorn should only start after consultation with a doctor or medical herbalist. Before using any herbal treatment that might affect the heart directly, I strongly recommend that the advice of a doctor or qualified herbal practitioner be sought. No treatment of heart problems should be undertaken without careful consideration, and this is unlikely to be achieved without training. I must emphasise that not following this advice could have serious consequences.

Houttuynia * *Houttuynia cordata*

History/traditional use

Houttuynia is native to Asia; in China it is known as Yu Xing Cao. In Japan the houttuynia plant is commonly called "*dokudami*" – "poison-blocking plant". It has been used since ancient times to clear poisons. The leaves have been shown to benefit the lungs and kidneys, to regulate blood glucose levels, and to reduce fever and infection.

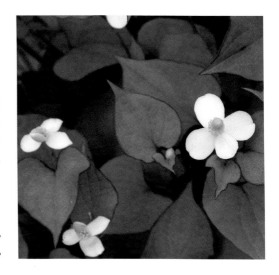

Action: Antiallergenic, anticancer, anti-inflammatory, antimicrobial, antioxidant, antitussive, antiviral, detoxicant, diuretic, hepatoprotective.

Modern use

Lyme disease and co-infections: Houttuynia is a fairly good broad-spectrum antiviral and antibacterial herb in that it reduces inflammation, lowers the cytokine cascade in cellular tissue, and stimulates the immune system. It has been shown to be of particular benefit to those who have resistant strains of Bartonella or biofilms affecting the oral cavity.

Herbalists Stephen Buhner, James Schaller, Lee Cowden, and Ying Zhang pioneered the use houttuynia, among other herbs, for co-infections such as herpes viruses, mycoplasma biofilms, and Bartonella.

Anti-allergic activity: Houttuynia has demonstrated anti-allergic activity by affecting mast cells, decreasing histamine release, and showing benefits for allergic conditions such as asthma and allergic rhinitis.

Women's health: The root is used in medicinal preparations as an emmenagogue; it can also bring on menstrual cycles where there is a delayed period.

Anti-inflammatory uses: Houttuynia is used for rheumatoid arthritis and for various inflammatory conditions of the chest, such as severe or acute respiratory syndromes. It improves oxyhaemoglobin saturation levels of the blood. It is being looked at as a potential inhibitor for severe acute respiratory syndrome (SARS) and coronavirus replication.

Houttuynia also shows strong antioxidant properties in mopping up free radicals.

Cultivation

Spread by rhizomes, this invasive plant is found throughout China and Eastern Asia. Striking leaves spread vigorously, creating a dense ground-cover in late spring or early summer. Likes moist ground, full sun to part shade. Grows well in a bog garden or a permanently moist border, as it can tolerate up to 5 cm of standing water.

Harvesting/foraging

The leaves and young shoots are harvested in the spring, when about 8 cm long. The fresh plant contains higher antiviral and antibacterial activity.

How to use

Decoction: 15–30 g dried leaf decoction or 30–50 g fresh decoction daily. Brief decoction in order not to inactivate antimicrobial activity.

Tincture: Fresh leaf: 20–60 drops, three times a day. It has a fishy smell, so smells and tastes best when mixed with other herbs.

Used as an antiviral: 5 ml tincture of the fresh leaf, three times a day.

Used against mycoplasma and Bartonella: 2.5 ml tincture of the fresh leaf, three times a day (Buhner).[35]

Wounds: *Paste:* mix a small amount of mashed fresh plant and apply to heal wounds.

Caution/contraindications

Avoid during pregnancy or when breast-feeding.

Japanese knotweed * *Fallopia japonica*

History/traditional use

Japanese knotweed, one of the most popular herbs in the Chinese pharmacopeia (and known as Hu Zhang), was introduced to the United Kingdom in 1825 as an ornamental shrub. Japanese knotweed, *Fallopia japonica*, has also been classified as *Polygonum cuspidatum* and *Reynoutria japonica*.

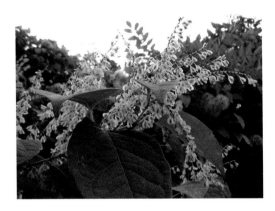

The Chinese use Japanese knotweed as a tonic to improve vitality and health and to treat fungal infections, burns, cardiovascular, respiratory, and neurodegenerative disorders, cancers, diabetes, and hair loss. It is a rich source of resveratrol, a powerful antioxidant.

Action: Analgesic, anticancer, antifungal, anti-inflammatory, antioxidative, anti-spirochete, antitussive, antiviral, astringent, capillary stimulant, cytokine modulator, diuretic, expectorant, immune modulator, immune stimulant, immunomodulator, laxative, neuroregenerative, phytoestrogenic, protects liver and central nervous system.

Modern use

Lyme disease: Japanese knotweed has a broad-spectrum antibacterial activity effective against spirochetes. It is one of the main ingredients in Buhner's Lyme disease protocol.[36] It is particularly useful in crossing the blood–brain barrier, reducing oxidative stress and inflammation in the brain.

Japanese knotweed is high in resveratrol. It shows significant results (*in vitro*) in reducing *Borrelia burgdorferi and B. garinii* biofilm and breaking down gram-positive and gram-negative bacteria.

Scientists have also found that emodin, a compound found in Japanese knotweed, improves immune function by increasing the production of natural killer cells, B cells, and T cells, and protects the liver and the brain from inflammation. Further studies indicate that Japanese knotweed could be used to reduce histamine and allergies.

Japanese knotweed can reduce Herxheimer reactions while protecting organs that have been damaged by the endotoxins and die-off from bacteria.

Antiviral: Resveratrol can suppress the viral replication and growth of a wide range of viruses, such as influenza type A, cytomegalovirus, ECHO virus, and herpes simplex. Emodin has also been shown to block the attachment of a virus to the host cell in SARS.

Antibacterial: Japanese knotweed is thought to be active against a wide range of bacteria by inhibiting bacterial DNA primase, an enzyme involved in replication – for example, in *E. coli*, streptococcus, and salmonella.

Over time, Japanese knotweed has been shown to break down biofilms in dental cavities; it is used as a mouthwash in Korea.

Cardiovascular – improves blood flow: Resveratrol acts as a vasodilator, lowers blood pressure, inhibits platelet aggregation, improves microcirculation, and enhances blood flow to the brain and other organs. It can reduce symptoms associated with the heart, such as shortness of breath, palpitations, lightheadedness.

Japanese knotweed's antioxidant properties have been shown to protect telomeres from damage. Telomeres sit at the end strand of our DNA, a bit like the plastic tips at the end of a shoelace. They gradually shrink with age. Stopping the ends fraying protects our genetic material. The telomeres affect the replicative life span and health of our cells.

The problem is that a stressful lifestyle can shrink these protective caps, making it increasingly likely for cells to die and stop dividing. The loss of cell power and growth accelerates the aging process. The shorter the telomeres, the more likely that the body will experience inflammation. The earlier this happens, the more likely we are to begin to suffer from ailments for which we may have a genetic predisposition.

Metabolism: Resveratrol has been used to influence energy restriction and therefore blood sugar control. It mimics a calorie restriction by increasing a cascade of events that ultimately increase mitochondrial function. This is a bit like a 2/5 diet restriction, where you restrict calories to 500–600 for two days, and then eat normally for 5 days. The benefits are claimed to be improved cognitive function and increased life span.

Cancer: The research suggests benefits in chemotherapy treatment. Japanese knotweed may curb the proliferation of breast and ovarian cancer.

Transcription factor NF-κB, a protein found in all cells, is critical for immunity and cell proliferation and is seen as a key regulator of inflammation in response to stressful stimuli; if unregulated, it can trigger the growth of cells and cancer.

Resveratrol also stimulates tumour suppressor proteins, which are important for DNA repair.

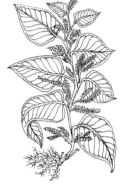

Neuroprotective effect: Japanese knotweed is thought to have a neuroprotective effect against neurotoxic substances. It may help people suffering from neurological damage – for example, in Alzheimer's disease – by decreasing the breakdown of acetylcholine. Scientists are also looking at the benefits of this plant in supporting people with Parkinson's by protecting dopamine neurons from damage, as well as protecting the brain from the damage caused by strokes and tissue ischemia. It also protects the brain against glutamate toxicity, especially where this involves memory loss and symptoms of chronic fatigue.[37]

Cultivation

Japanese knotweed is an invasive species, and it is illegal to grow it. Grows quickly along the edges of fields, waterways, and roads, with a particular fondness for disturbed areas or wasteland. It is considered a gardener's nightmare, a noxious weed, with eradication programmes being set up all over the world, as it is difficult to get rid of and can break through concrete. In Japan and China, Japanese knotweed is managed by natural predators like insects and fungi that control its spread. In the United Kingdom, homeowners who allow Japanese knotweed to grow could be fined £2,500 under new rules that class failing to control the problem plant as "antisocial behaviour". If a company fails to act, they could face a £20,000 fine. The root must be dug up, bagged, and disposed of properly to prevent further spread. Harvesting from the wild is not recommended, for the reasons mentioned above, particularly as the knotweed may have been sprayed with toxic pesticides.

Harvesting/foraging

The leaf is edible, and in China it is harvested in early spring and eaten like asparagus.

How to use

Often used for 12 months, or until symptoms resolve.

Decoction: Add 25 g root to 1 litre water, simmer for 20 minutes, and drink throughout the day.

Tincture: tinctured root, ½ tsp, two to three times a day.

Raw powder: 1 tsp raw powder can be added to smoothies or liquid and taken three times a day.

Capsules: 500 mg, one to three times a day, slowly building up to 3 capsules, four times a day; 9–15 grams of whole herb can be taken a day.

Extract: 5:1 concentrates = 1–3 capsules a day.

Caution/contraindications

Very few studies on resveratrol have been conducted in humans. Doctors cannot make claims or confirm any benefits. However, resveratrol may interact with blood thinners and lower blood sugar levels. Other symptoms may include dry mouth, nausea, vomiting, abdominal pain, a bitter taste in the mouth, and diarrhoea.

The leaf contains oxalic acid and should be avoided in high doses if there is a history of kidney stones and arthritis. Less oxalic acid is found in the root.

History/traditional use

Milk thistle, which is a member of the *Asteraceae* family, is known for improving liver function, especially when toxins are involved. It has been used for over 2,000 years to treat liver, kidney, and gall bladder disorders. It was thought to cure rabies and was used as an antimalarial. The leaves and stems have been used in cooking. A related species is *Carduus marianus*.

Action: Anti-inflammatory, antioxidant, antiviral, galactagogic (increases breast milk production), hepatoprotective.

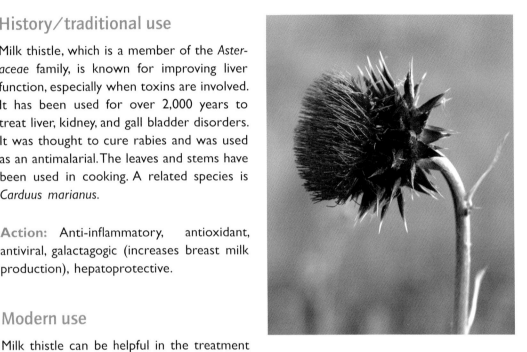

Modern use

Milk thistle can be helpful in the treatment of Lyme disease, as it can help to reduce cell damage, toxins, viruses, and inflammation. Not regulating glucose levels can impair immune function and the body's ability to get rid of bacteria. Regulating sugar levels could therefore also have significant benefits in supporting people with Lyme disease.

Inflammation: Milk thistle's polyphenolic flavonoids, first found in the seeds, have antioxidant properties. They break down to silymarin, which has been shown to have anti-inflammatory properties by blocking inflammation pathways.

Immunity: Milk thistle supports liver function. The liver plays a vital role as part of the immune system: it is the first line of defence. Kupffer cells found in the liver are macrophages, which defend the body against blood-borne disease.

It has also been shown to block NF-κB – a protein, found in all cells, that controls transcription of DNA – and can reduce inflammation. This protein is critical for immunity and cell proliferation and is seen as a key regulator of inflammation in response to stressful stimuli such as a viral infection.

Liver: Some co-infections, including viruses, can cause an impaired bile flow or elevate liver enzymes. When this happens, the liver is unable to keep up with the filtering of bilirubin when the red cells die. Liver support therefore is crucial.

The main extract in milk thistle that contributes to treating liver disease is silymarin. Silymarin is collectively made up of the flavonolignans silybin, silychristin, and silidianin. These extracts have hepatoprotective, anti-inflammatory, and antioxidant regenerative properties.[38] Silymarin enhances glutathione production, an antioxidant that protects against cell damage. As glutathione is an essential component for detoxifying, it is easy to see why it is a popular over-the-counter hangover cure.[39] Milk thistle is therefore a good herb of choice for people who are chemically sensitive or are experiencing Herxheimer reactions.

Diabetes: Milk thistle is a beneficial herb to consider in regulating blood glucose levels. In a random double-blind trial, 51 Type-2 diabetic patients with non-alcoholic fatty liver disease (often associated with metabolic syndrome) received, in addition to their metformin, 600 mg milk thistle extract a day for 4 months. The fasting blood sugar in the milk thistle group showed significant reduction when compared to the placebo group.[40] This makes it a useful herb in addition to metformin in improving sugar control and improving Lyme disease outcomes.

Anaesthesia: Kerry Bone found high doses of milk thistle extract for 3 weeks before and 4–8 weeks after general anaesthesia to be greatly beneficial in minimising its toxic effect.[41]

Cultivation

Native to the Mediterranean area, milk thistle has naturalised itself world-wide on wasteland. It grows to 60–120 cm tall and has alternate leaves and prickles, with milk-white veins on the leaves. The flowers are purple and spiky, producing black shiny seeds, crowned in their white fluffy pappus. Each flower can produce about 190 seeds.

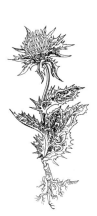

Harvesting/foraging

Seeds are harvested from July onwards, into the autumn.

How to use

Tincture: 1:5 or 1:3 strength, 45% ethanol tincture or seeds, 2–4 ml, three times a day.

Caution/contraindications

Silymarin has a good safety record, with only rare gastrointestinal effects. Possible drug interaction with cytochrome enzymes, so check with health practitioner if on medication.[42]

Motherwort   ✳   *Leonurus cardiaca*

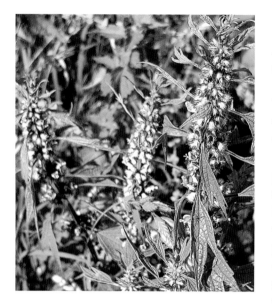

History/traditional use

An old saying goes: "Drink motherwort tea and live to be a source of continuous astonishment and frustration to your wanting heir!" The specific botanical name for this plant, which is a member of the mint or labiate family, refers to its association with the heart. Motherwort is one of the best remedies for palpitations associated with a sense of fear and raised pulse rate, its action having a relaxing, calming, and stabilising effect. It has been traditionally used to treat tachycardia, anxiety, palpitations in hyperthyroid conditions, and cardiac debility. Also used as a womb remedy for painful periods, mostly those associated with tension, anxiety, or fibroids; for heavy periods; and during the menopause.

Action: Anti-arrhythmic, anti-inflammatory, antispasmodic, cardiac tonic, sedative.

Modern use

More recently, motherwort has been shown to have anti-inflammatory properties. Pharmacology studies have confirmed its antibacterial, antioxidant, anti-inflammatory, and analgesic activity.[43] It has higher antioxidant properties than hawthorn and ginkgo and can protect the mitochondria of a cell.

Lyme disease: Motherwort helps with many cardiac, mitochondrial, and inflammatory aspects of Lyme disease.

Inflammation: Ursolic acid – a compound found in the aerial part of motherwort – has an antioxidant, antimicrobial, and anti-inflammatory effect. By inhibiting both COX-2 and 5-LOX pathways, it can further reduce inflammation of the brain, which can cause pressure in the brain.

Ursolic acid has been shown to be protective against ischemic injury in mice after a stroke, by antioxidant and anti-inflammatory action.[44] Buhner uses motherwort to help support mitochondrial integrity, "especially where there is ischemia reperfusion induced by mitochondria dysfunction in the brain".[45]

Cultivation

Grows on wasteground and roadsides and in hedgerows throughout Europe, Asia, and North America, though avoiding the very northern latitudes; found throughout Britain. Grows 16–200 cm tall. Coarsely toothed, very thick square stem, 5–7 lobes, opposite leaves. Flowers in each whorl, with pink petals; they have an unpleasant odour.

Harvesting/foraging

Harvested between July and September. Chop down just before flowering and place in a shredder, or cut up. Turn into a tincture when fresh.

How to use

Infusion: Herbal tea: 8–14 g a day; 30 g in half a litre of water.

Tincture: 1:3 strength, 45% ethanol tincture, 2–5 ml, three times a day.

Capsules: 100–200 mg (use higher doses of 400–500 mg if used alone).

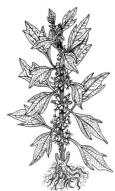

Caution/contraindications

Avoid in pregnancy: uterine stimulant yet mild emmenagogue due to high tannin levels, could cause bleeding. But it has been used toward the end of labour, to reduce anxiety, improve effective contractions, and promote a speedy delivery.

May lower blood pressure.

Olive ❊ *Olea europaea*

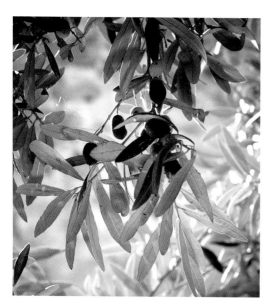

History/traditional use

The olive tree, originating in Mediterranean countries, dating back over 6,000 years is rich in nutrients. A symbol of peace, it was used to make crowns in ancient Greece. Olive oil is traditionally used as a cardiac tonic or a liver aid, and for lowering cholesterol and sugar levels and reducing blood pressure; it has antimicrobial benefits.

Action: Anti-arthritic, antibacterial, antifungal, antioxidant, antiparasitic, antiseptic, antiviral, astringent, diuretic, hypotensive, immune-boosting.

Modern use

Anti-inflammatory: Oleocanthal, a phytonutrient found in olive leaf, has anti-inflammatory effects, reducing brain and joint inflammation.

Scientific investigations suggest that it has properties similar to ibuprofen. Daily intake has a cumulative effect. Studies show that, taken 2 weeks prior to periods, it can significantly reduce period pain.[46]

Cardiovascular tonic: Olive oil inhibits platelet activity, which can, in the long term, reduce the risk of arteriosclerosis. It oxygenates and improves blood flow, not only to the brain, but to the liver and pancreas as well. Its antioxidant ability is higher than that of vitamin E.

By reducing prostaglandin synthesis and improving antioxidant enzymes, it can help to reduce swelling. It can be seen as protective for the brain, heart, liver, and pancreas.

Antimicrobial: The leaf has a variety of antimicrobial activity. Buhner's protocol to reduce mycoplasma infections infuses the leaf in oil.[47]

There is some evidence to suggest that extracts of olive leaf inhibit the herpes and Coxsackie virus and the staphylococcus and *E. coli* bacteria.

Digestion: Olive oil has a positive effect on the gut microbiota, protecting the lining of the digestive system, regulating blood sugar levels, and protecting the liver from hepatotoxins.

Cultivation

Native to the Mediterranean region, the olive is now cultivated widely all over the world.

Harvesting/foraging

Olive fruit are harvested when ripe in the autumn; leaves can be harvested all year round or be picked up freely in the spring, when the leaves are being pruned and left on the ground.

How to use

Leaf infusion: Steep 1 heaped tsp leaf in 1 cup of boiling water, three times a day.

Tincture: 5 ml can be taken two to three times a day, for its antimicrobial activity or to reduce high blood pressure.

Capsules: Take after food to increase absorption. Capsules can vary – a standardised extract of 250 mg Oleuropein and 250 mg olive leaf can be taken: 1 capsule, three times a day.

Oil: Infusing cold-pressed virgin olive oil with olive leaf can be used after 2 weeks. Use liberally in your diet.

Evidence suggests an infused olive leaf and oil – e.g., 25 ml of olive oil a day – can reduce pain and is part of Buhner's mycoplasma protocol.[48]

Infused oil: Fill half a jar with leaf and cover with oil – oil to come at least 5 cm above the leaf, so that no leaf is showing; place in a warm place for 2 weeks, or, to speed up the process, place ingredients in a slow cooker and gently warm for 3–4 hours; once done, squeeze the oil and rebottle to use as needed.

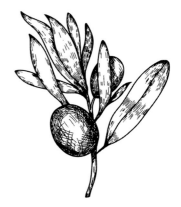

Caution/contraindications

Can have a laxative effect. Monitor blood pressure, as it can have a lowering effect.

Pomegranate * *Punica granatum*

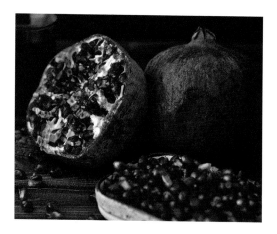

History/traditional use

Pomegranate has had a prominent role as a healing food throughout Mediterranean and Middle Eastern history. It dates back to biblical times and was used as a symbol in religious ceremonies.

Action: Anti-Alzheimer's, antidiabetic, anti-inflammatory, antimicrobial, antioxidant, antitumour, antiviral, cardioprotective.

Modern use

Cardiovascular health: Pomegranate is high in vitamins A, C, and E. Its flavanols make it particularly useful in protecting the heart and in treating headaches and muscle stiffness.

Gut health: Extracts of pomegranate can help with increasing liver enzymes and detoxification pathways.

Eating pomegranate fruit or using it as a mouthwash can help reduce bacteria and improve antioxidant effect around the teeth and gums.

Friendly gut bacteria of *Bifidobacterium breve* and *B. infantis* are increased when consuming pomegranate.

Lyme disease and co-infections: Pomegranate has been reported to improve cognitive functions and power and to reduce inflammatory conditions such as arthritic-type symptoms, neurodegenerative disease, and fibromyalgia, reducing stress levels and symptoms of fatigue.

Buhner uses pomegranate juice as part of his mycoplasma and Bartonella protocol.[49]

It has an additional benefit in that it increases the effectiveness of drugs such as ampicillin, chloramphenicol, gentamicin, and tetracycline.

Cultivation

Iran, India, and China are the major exporters of pomegranates, which grow best where there are long hot summers. Pomegranates prefer a warm and sunny location with well-drained soil, and they can be grown in a greenhouse or against a south-facing wall to provide extra protection from the cold. Too much rain or a winter freeze can damage the plant, and drought can affect yield.

Harvesting/foraging

The fruit is harvested between September and February in the northern hemisphere. In the southern hemisphere it is harvested between March and May.

Fruit, seed, juice, and rind are used for malarial *Plasmodium falciparum*.

How to use

Eating pomegranate in salads or drinking pomegranate juice daily can have an immune-boosting effect.

Juice: 220 ml of pomegranate juice every 3 hours during a mycoplasma infection; 200 ml or 225 g a day for 1 month can improve memory performance.

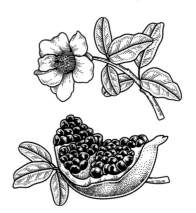

Caution/contraindications

May lower blood pressure, but is mostly safe, unless taken with a lot of medication. Sensitivity to this plant is rare.

Rock rose * *Cistus incanus*

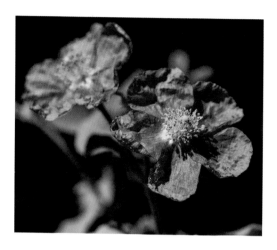

History/traditional use

The rock rose is a shrub native to the Mediterranean region. In traditional medicine the plant has been widely used for its antibacterial, anti-inflammatory, and antiviral properties. In some cultures it was used as a herbal remedy for various ailments, such as coughs, colds, digestive issues, rheumatism, gout, skin disorders, fevers, and diarrhoea.

Actions: Adaptogenic, antibacterial, antifungal, antioxidant, antiviral, immune-modulating.

Modern use

Dietrich Klinghardt uses wild rock rose as part of his protocol for treating cancers triggered by retroviruses and Lyme disease. In his clinic he uses rock rose to disrupt biofilms, to reduce symptoms of chronic Lyme disease and Epstein-Barr virus infection, and for its retroviral activity, which, he found, can be detected using the Autonomic Response Technique (ART).[50]

Immunity: Some studies have indicated that rock rose has the potential to inhibit the replication of certain retroviruses, such as the human immunodeficiency virus (HIV). Additionally, extracts of rock rose applied to the skin reduce redness and inflammation associated with psychological stress, with potential anti-aging benefits. However, it is important to note that the results of these studies are still preliminary: more research is needed to fully understand the antiviral and healing activity of rock rose and its potential as a treatment for infections.

Cultivation

The rock rose is a drought-tolerant and heat-loving plant that thrives in well-drained soils with full sun exposure. It prefers a warm and dry climate and is typically found in rocky or sandy soils near the coast. The plant is hardy and can tolerate salt spray, making it well suited for coastal gardens.

Rock rose should be watered sparingly and only when the soil is completely dry, as too much moisture can lead to root rot.

Harvesting/foraging

Harvest in the summer, when the plant is in full bloom and the essential oils in the leaves and flowers are at their highest concentration. Pruning should be done after flowering to maintain a neat appearance and encourage new growth.

How to use

Infusion: Bring 1–2 teaspoons of dried leaves and flowers per cup of water slowly to a boil, and simmer for 5 minutes with a lid on; 6–8 cups a day of rock rose infusion, sweetened with Stevia, can be taken each day. The tea can be re-brewed 3–4 times.

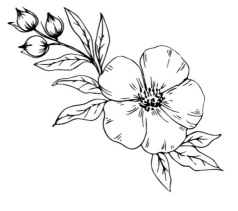

Caution/contraindications

There are few reported side effects associated with the use of rock rose.

Sage   ✳   *Salvia officinalis*
Red sage   ✳   *Salvia miltiorrhiza*

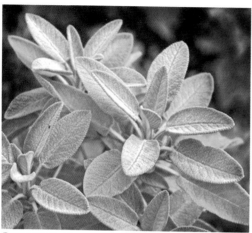
Common sage

History/traditional use

There are many species of sage that are used in herbal medicine. The two most often used are sage (*Salvia officinalis,* also known as common or culinary sage) and red sage (*Salvia miltiorrhiza,* also known as Chinese sage, or Danshen). They belong to the same genus, Salvia, and both species have been used for centuries by indigenous peoples for their medicinal properties: to reduce inflammatory diseases, neurodegenerative diseases, menopause and cardiovascular disorders. Although they share some similarities in terms of their medicinal properties, they are used to treat different conditions and have different active compounds.

Common sage is used in cooking and as a natural remedy for digestive issues, sore throats, indigestion, and menopausal symptoms. Red sage is used to treat a number of ailments by improving circulation but is mainly used to treat cardiovascular disease.

Action: *Common sage:* antibacterial, antifungal, anti-inflammatory, antimicrobial, antiparasitic, antiseptic, antispasmodic, phytoestrogenic.
Red sage: Anti-atherosclerosis, anticoagulant, anti-inflammatory, antioxidant, calmative, endothelial protective, oestrogenic, vasodilatory.

Modern use

Circulation: Red sage is used in traditional Chinese medicine to improve circulation and blood flow in reproductive and cardiovascular conditions improve blood flow, while reduce platelet clotting time. It is often used in treating conditions such as chest pain angina, hypertension, and irregular menstruation.

One of the many active compounds, known as tanshinones, has been found to have anti-inflammatory and antioxidant effects.

Some studies have suggested that when treating babesiosis, red sage may have a protective effect, preventing the destruction of red blood cells. *In vitro* and *in vivo* studies have suggested that the compounds in red sage, including tanshinones, danshensu, and cryptotanshinone, have anti-Babesia activity by inhibiting the growth and replication of the parasites.

Its antimicrobial properties against Babesia and Ehrlichia, and protective and strengthening effect on the liver, spleen, lungs, heart, and bones, show promise in supporting people with Lyme disease.

Immune system: Some preliminary studies suggest that the compounds found in common sage have antifungal and antimicrobial properties, which may be effective against the bacteria that causes Lyme disease. Its antiparasitic properties have been used in the treatment of malaria, but it is not well studied for Babesia.

Research has suggested that the compounds found in common sage, such as rosmarinic acid, have anti-inflammatory and antioxidant properties.

Gut health: Common sage has been found to have potential effects on the vagus nerve, which is the longest cranial nerve and has a wide range of functions including controlling the digestive system and regulating the immune response. (The vagus nerve is discussed in greater detail in chapter 7.)

Several studies have investigated the effects of red sage on gut health and biofilm formation, in particular the regulation of Lactobacillus and bifidobacterium. Red sage has been found to support the development of healthy biofilm in the gut while also having the potential to slowly disrupt pathogenic biofilm. It is worth mentioning that many of these studies were done either in *in vitro* or with animal models, so more research is needed to confirm these findings in humans.

Mood: The antimicrobial and anti-inflammatory properties of common sage improve cognitive function and memory, which is particularly useful for those suffering from brain fog, sore throats, and hot flushes. Red sage is considered as a calming herb, combining to receptors sites, similar to benzodiazepines.

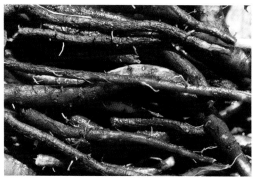

Red sage root

Its mild sedative activity can help those who are suffering from stress and anxiety without the habit-forming side effect of benzodiazepines.[51]

Both species contain phytoestrogen, which has a hormonal mimicking effect, which is why they are both commonly used for menopausal conditions such as hot flushes; this oestrogenic effect may contribute to reducing inflammation in the body.

However, more research is needed to confirm these findings and to understand the potential effectiveness of common sage in supporting those with Lyme disease. It is important to reiterate that the use of herbs as a treatment for any of the conditions mentioned in this book should be done under the supervision of a qualified healthcare provider or doctor.

Cultivation

Both species are perennials. Common sage, which is native to the Mediterranean region, is widely cultivated in many parts of the world. It enjoys moist soil and a warm, sheltered position in full sun, although it can handle dappled shade.

Red sage is native to China and the southeastern United States. It enjoys well-draining soil, with about half a day of sunlight. It is hardy to approximately −10 °C (14 °F).

Harvesting/foraging

Collect seeds or grow from cuttings taken in spring. Leaves can be harvested May to June, best after the second year of growth and onwards. Sage should be cut frequently, especially in spring, to ensure a good healthy growth.

How to use

Common sage

Infusion: 1–4 g per day of dried herb.

Tablet: 300 mg dose is effective.

Tincture: 1.5 strength, 2–4 ml a day.

Gargle or tea: I tsp. dried herb.

Sage and myrrh toothpaste

 I tbsp common sage
 I tsp salt
 5 drops of myrrh

• Grind sage and salt together in a pestle and mortar. Add the myrrh and mix well.

• Brush on your gums using a toothbrush; do not swallow.

Red sage root

Tincture: I.5 strength, 2–4 ml a day.

Decoction: 9–15 g daily dose.

Caution/contraindications

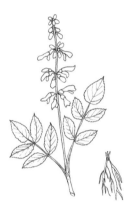

Sage species are generally recognized as having a safe status. However, common sage is contraindicated in pregnancy as it can bring on delayed bleeding, or when breast feeding as it may reduce lactation. Large quantities of thujone oil extracted from the plant can cause harm to the central nervous system.

Do not use red sage with medication that has a blood-thinning effect.

Sarsaparilla * *Smilax glabra*

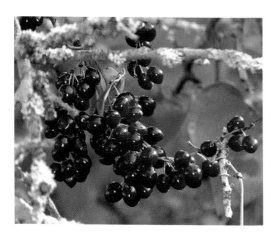

History/traditional use

Sarsaparilla, also known as smilax, and in China as Tu Fu Ling, has been used by Native American people for thousands of years to lower inflammation and raise immunity against bacteria and fungi. It has a history in the treatment for allergies, painful joints, and kidney, skin, respiratory conditions, and syphilis.

Action: Antibacterial, anti-inflammatory, antiparasitic, binds to endotoxins, blood cleanser, hepatoprotective, immunomodulator, neuroprotective.

Main constituents: Sarsaparilla contains plant steroids and saponins, which enhance the bioavailability of other drugs and phytochemicals.

Modern use

Skin: Sarsaparilla contains plant steroids and saponins, which enhance the bioavailability of other drugs and phytochemicals. Steroidal saponins are anti-inflammatory chemical compounds with antimicrobial properties that reduce skin disorders such as psoriasis, acne, eczema, leprosy, and gout.

Hormones: Steroidal saponins have been used to mimic and restore hormone balance, and in the treatment of menopausal symptoms and low libido in both men and women. Beneficial in the treatment of diabetes and regulating blood glucose levels.

Immunity: As an immunomodulator, Sarsaparilla appears to down-regulate autoimmune disorders and stimulate specific immune responses to pathogens. Because of its antimicrobial and anti-inflammatory effects, it has been used to reduce respiratory symptoms, inhibit cough reflexes, break down mucus, and ease sore throats and inflamed nasal passages. It works in synergy with other herbs, improving their activity. There is some evidence to suggest that the hepatoprotective effect not only protects the liver from chemical damage caused by pathogens, it can also stabilise liver enzyme levels, making it a valuable herb for liver and gallbladder problems.

Lyme disease: Around the sixteenth century, sarsaparilla was brought to Europe as a treatment for syphilis and leptospirosis, both of which are caused by spirochete bacteria.

Sarsaparilla is capable of enhancing the activity of herbs and binding endotoxins; it can help with symptoms of Herxheimer reaction. As it can cross the blood–brain barrier, it can reduce cognitive problems associated with Lyme disease.

Joints: Sarsaparilla has also been used for painful joints and arthritis, as well as urination and liver, gallbladder, and digestive disorders, so has found its way into many Lyme protocols.

Cultivation

Sarsaparilla is a brambled, woody vine that can reach almost 50 m in length. There are over 350 species of sarsaparilla, native, variously, to Jamaica, the Caribbean, South America, Mexico, and Central America.

It is an invasive vine plant. Seed can be planted in the autumn; germination is best after a freeze.

Harvesting/foraging

Sarsaparilla is a climbing vine covered in prickles, so wear gloves. Follow the vine back to the root. Dig up in the autumn to harvest.

How to use

Sarsaparilla is used in various ways in Latin America to create fermented beverages and snacks.

Capsules: 425–500 mg, one to three times a day, for 8–12 months.

High doses are recommended for 2 months or while experiencing Herxheimer reactions.

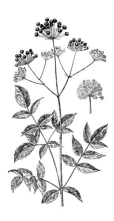

Tincture: 1:3 strength, 45% alcohol, 2–4 ml, two to three times a day, in a little water.

If symptoms lessen, reduce the amount of herbs.

Caution/contraindications

Side effects have rarely been reported. Because studies are limited, avoid if pregnant.

Large doses can irritate the digestive tract and speed the elimination of medication.

Siberian ginseng * *Eleutherococcus senticosus*

History/traditional use

Siberian ginseng has traditionally been used in China and Russia to improve general wellbeing, strengthen the spleen, and nourish the kidney. It has also been used as a rejuvenating tonic by the elderly or sick. In the 1970s, the Russians used this herb in preparing for the Olympic games to strengthen and improve stamina and when suffering from muscle pain.

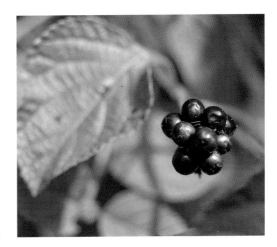

Action: Adaptogenic, anti-arrhythmic, antibacterial, antifungal, antiviral, immunomodulator, mild stimulant/tonic, regulates uterine function.

Modern use

Siberian ginseng can help with the exhaustion aspects of Lyme disease.

Fatigue: Siberian ginseng has been found helpful for overcoming exhaustion in cases of chronic fatigue. Siberian ginseng was also found to boost mitochondrial function in the cardiac muscles, increasing oxygenation of organs and energy levels, improving stamina and cognitive function, normalising blood sugar levels, strengthening the body's resistance to daily stress, and aiding recovery after surgery.

Immunity: Siberian ginseng has been shown to improve healing and to boost the immune system. It does this by enhancing the activity of T helper cells and natural killer cells. It is being considered in cancer therapies, as it has been shown to reduce chromosomal mutations.

Siberian ginseng's antimicrobial effects have been shown to stimulate antiviral activity and reduce inflammation by inhibiting COX-2 pathways.

Cultivation

Native to northern China, Korea, Japan, and south-eastern Russia, ginseng grows in mountainous areas in full sun or partial shade. A small, woody shrub, it likes sand and humus in soil. It is considered difficult to germinate: some growers incubate seeds and soil in a fridge for 10–24 months to get seed to sprout. It can be invasive, given the right conditions.

Harvesting/foraging

Harvest roots after third year of growth.

How to use

Decoction: 1–4 g a day.

Tincture: 1:5 strength, 2 ml, three times a day for conditions like chronic fatigue; 1:1 strength, 5 ml, three times a day for 30 days for chronic conditions.

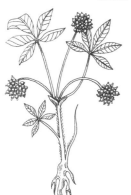

Capsules: 2 capsules, 450 g, four times a day, for 8–12 months. In Chinese medicine, the dose can vary, 4–20 g a day.

Caution/contraindications

May cause insomnia and hyperactivity (especially when taken with caffeine). High doses may increase blood pressure. Avoid with high blood pressure, anticoagulants (blood thinners). Avoid if pregnant or breastfeeding. Generally not taken for more than 3 months without a break or in acute phase of infection.

Silver birch * *Betula alba*

History/traditional use

A tree known for its silvery-white thin bark, peeling off in layers. Found in woodlands throughout Britain and the northern hemisphere.

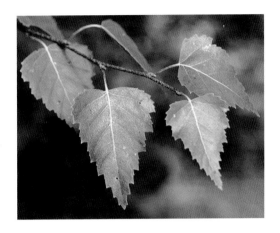

Action: Anti-arthritic, anti-inflammatory, antiseptic, digestive, diuretic, liver tonic, slight sedative.

Modern use

Sugar alternative: The rationing of sugar in Europe in the Second World War led to research to find sugar substitutes. Xylitol was one of these: sugar alcohol synthesised from the birch tree using chemicals. It is slightly sweeter than sugar, with 40% fewer calories, its antibacterial properties making it a chewing gum popular among dentists to prevent tooth decay.[52] This may be a particularly beneficial alternative to sugar for those with diabetes or who want to lose weight or those with metabolic disorders.

Anti-inflammatory: The essential oil, which is found in the bark, is related to the salicylates found in willow and oil of wintergreen; due to its aspirin-like properties it is used both internally and externally, for arthritic conditions and for skin problems. For external use the sap is most convenient, although a poultice of the leaves can be placed around an inflamed joint.

Immunity: Betulinic acid, found in silver birch, has been shown to have a beneficial effect on the immune system. Research shows that it has antiviral,[53] antiparasitic,[54] antifungal,[55] and anticarcinogenic activities[56] and has strong antimicrobial activity with the inhibition of *E. coli.*, chlamydia pneumonia, and staphylococcus.[57]

Waterworks: The leaves have an antiseptic, anti-inflammatory, diuretic action and an antimicrobial effect on the urinary system.

Cultivation

A fast-growing tree, silver birch is found in woodlands throughout Britain and the whole northern hemisphere. The leaves are broadly ovate, tapering to a fine point, smooth-toothed and shiny, but with minute glandular dots when young. The male catkins droop, 2–5 cm long; the female, on short stalks, can be up to 15 cm long.

Harvesting/foraging

Young leaves are collected and dried in April and May, the sap, and the leaf buds in spring; the bark and branches are harvested in the autumn. The Russians preserve the buds in vodka as a treatment for inflammatory conditions.

Sap collection: Sap is obtained by inserting a tube into holes bored in the trunk and collecting in a vessel for up to 2 days, preserving the fluid in an alcohol–water mixture (adding 1 part of vodka or similar to 3 parts of sap). A dose of 2 tsp three times per day is recommended. To infuse the leaves, add a pinch of bicarbonate of soda to each pint to aid extraction of the active constituents. The dose of infusion is the same as for other remedies in this book.

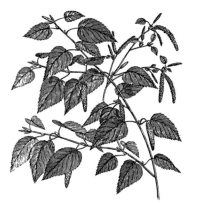

How to use

Infusion: 2–4 g, three times a day, of birch leaf infusion as a tea; maximum dose 12 g.

Decoction: Made from the small branches and bark, boiled for 15 minutes.[58]

Caution/contraindications

People allergic to birch pollen and those with salicylic sensitivity or oedema where there is reduced cardiac or kidney function should avoid this plant; also contraindicated during pregnancy, due to lack of research on its safety.

Sweet wormwood   *   *Artemisia annua*

History/traditional use

Sweet wormwood has been used for the last 2,000 years to treat fevers, parasites, nausea, and headaches. Reference has been found in an ancient Chinese text (Ge Hong's *Zhouhou Beiji Fang* [*Handbook of Prescriptions for Emergency*]) dating back to the Eastern Jin Dynasty, 317–420 AD) regarding its use as treatment for malaria. In 2001 WHO recommended the use of artemisinin-based combination therapies for malaria. Other forms, including tea made from the plant's leaves, have appeared as antimalarial remedies. A related and widely used species in Africa is African wormwood (*A. afra.*)

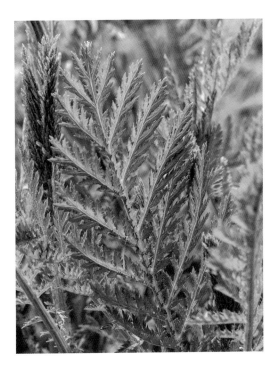

Action: Anti-arrhythmic, antibacterial, anti-fungal, anti-inflammatory, anti-parasitic, antiviral, mild laxative, regulates uterine function.

Modern use

Other species of Artemisia are used in the drinks industry, to make Southern Comfort from southernwood (*Artemisia abrotanum*) or absinthe from *Artemisia absinthium.*

Artemisinin is effective against multi–drug-resistant malaria; it is known to act on *P. falciparum*, the Plasmodium species that causes cerebral malaria. The clinical efficacy of this drug and its derivatives is demonstrated by immediate and rapid reduction of parasitemia following treatment.

Artemisinin has also been used in the treatment of Borrelia and of Lyme co-infections by Babesia, Ehrlichia, Bartonella, and mycoplasma.

Antiviral properties: Artemisinin's antiviral action is particularly useful in cases of herpes virus and other parasites.[59]

Anticancer properties: Artemisinin can bolster the effect of anticancer drugs by disrupting key biological functions, causing cancer cells to die.[60]

Cultivation

Sweet wormwood is native to temperate Asia. It is a short-day annual. It prefers cold temperatures in semi-shady woodlands and grows at high altitudes in damp areas of Korea, Japan, and China.

Its stem is erect brownish or violet brown. The plant itself is hairless and naturally grows 30–100 cm tall, although in cultivation it is possible for plants to reach a height of 200 cm.

Sow indoors in spring, 6–8 weeks before the last frost, or directly into the soil when all risk of frost has passed. Sow thinly, and thin out seedlings as required.

Mainly cultivated in temperate climates, at high altitudes.

Harvesting/foraging

The leaves are harvested in the summer, before the plant comes into flower, and dried for later use.

How to use

Sweet wormwood is more effective at a lower alcohol concentration.

Infusion: Simmer 4.5–9 g herbs to 1 litre of boiling water; allow to steep for 15 minutes.

Capsules: 800–1,200 daily for 7 days; this may correlate with the parasite causing symptoms around the moon cycles. For malaria, Day 1 dose: 500–100 mg; Day 2–4 dose: 4–5 mg a day. Repeat again in 2 weeks.

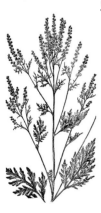

Tincture: 30% alcohol; dosage recommendation is 30 drops, 3 times a day, before food, 1–3 ml a day, for 5–7 days for a parasite infection, then have a break; you may benefit by repeating this once a month.

Caution/contraindications

Avoid if allergic or sensitive to the Artemisia or the wormwood family. Do not use if pregnant, breastfeeding, or have stomach or intestinal ulcers. Do not use for long periods.

Teasel ❊ *Dipsacus sativus*

History/traditional use

There are records of teasel being used in Chinese medicine for jaundice, to promote circulation, and to soothe sore and stiff joints, particularly the knees. It has traditionally been used to treat bladder infections. Teasel was used to tease and comb wool fibres in the textile industry or put in front of mice holes to stop the mice coming out.

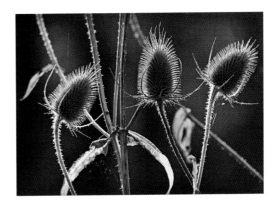

Action: Anti-arthritic, anti-inflammatory, antimicrobial, antioxidant, immunomodulatory activity.

Modern use

Lyme disease: Mathew Wood, a homeopath from the United States, uses this plant a lot to support people with Lyme disease. He uses the root and says:

> Teasel is excellent for chronic inflammation of the muscles, with limitation of movement and great pain. . . . Teasel is well indicated in chronic cases where a person becomes arthritic, the muscles all over are stiff and sore and they are eventually incapacitated.[61]

He describes it as easing pain where there has been stiffness and bruising, especially in the knee and lower back.

Other studies conducted on extracts from the leaf of *Dipsacus* species – *D. fullonum*, also known as wild teasel, or *D. sylvestris* – showed significant antimicrobial effects *in vitro* on *B. burgdorferi*.[62]

Little research is available about the precise biochemical mechanisms behind the effects of this plant; however, when I take it out of a tincture blend, my clients notice their joints aching more.

Other uses

▹ For structural repair, especially of connective tissue and bone.
▹ To alleviate muscle pain.
▹ For gut health: the inulin found in teasel root acts like a probiotic.
▹ As a diuretic.
▹ To increase circulation, and improve detoxification.
▹ To strengthens the knees and back.

Cultivation

Teasel is a wild growing, well distributed, and popular butterfly plant native to Europe, Asia, and northern Africa. You cannot mistake this biennial plant. The underside of the leaf is spiky on the main rib: in the wild, rainwater can collect in this receptacle. In the second year the egg-shaped flower heads, with purple, dark pink, or lavender petals, later dry, forming beautifully spiky seed heads.

Harvesting/foraging

Grows in open spaces and prefers full sunlight. You can find this plant by its giant rosette of leaves, which hug the ground during the first year of growth. The leaf, which has spikes on the underside, can be harvested from June to August, just before flowering.

Harvest the root after the first frost in the plant's first year.

How to use

Teasel root can be used in a tea (drink three times a day) or for making vinegar, glyceride, or tinctures.[63]

Decoction: The Chinese use the root: up to 6–12 g a day; can be simmered for 20 minutes, then drunk throughout the day.

Tincture: Leaf or root, 1:3 strength 45% alcohol, 2–10 drops just twice a day, for 1–3 months.

How to make a glycerite

▹ Dilute the glycerin with distilled water, 3 parts glycerin to 1 part water. To extend preservation time: 2 parts glycerin, 1 part water, 1 part alcohol.
▹ Fill the jar to 2/3 with fresh herb/root, or 1/2 the jar with dried herb/root.

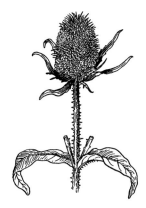

- Pour the glycerin + water into the jar to cover the herb and/or root.
- Leave in dry dark place for 6–8 weeks; shake the jar every couple of days.
- Strain and use.

Caution/contraindications

No toxic effects have been reported.

Wireweed   *   *Sida acuta*

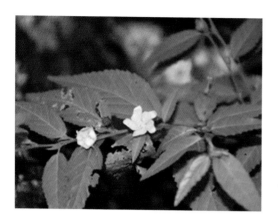

History/traditional use

Sida acuta, commonly known as wireweed, is widely used in Ayurvedic medicine for the treatment of fevers, urinary disorders, and digestive complaints by protecting the stomach lining, and thus having an antiulcer effect. It is traditionally used for malaria, anaemia, headache, fever, toothache, sore gums, arthritis, and diarrhoea and to regulate blood glucose levels. The Chinese consider it a useful remedy for depression, urinary stones, syphilitic effects on the skin, and respiratory infections. In Nicaragua and India it has been used for venereal disease and painful swellings of the testicles. Wireweed is believed to have originated in Central America,

Action: Adaptogenic, analgesic, antifungal, anti-inflammatory, antimicrobial, antioxidant, antiprotozoal, diuretic, hepatoprotective.

Modern use

Antimicrobial: Due to its broad-spectrum antibacterial, protective effect on red blood cells and on the liver and its antimicrobial properties, it is used against Babesia, Bartonella, and mycoplasma.

Wireweed has anti-inflammatory properties, strengthens the immune system, and stimulates glutathione production, which protects the red blood cells from damage caused by Bartonella bacteria.

Cryptolepine is an alkaloid isolated from both wireweed and Ghanaian quinine, which may be responsible for inhibiting the mechanism of parasite survival. This activity also has a beneficial effect in reducing some of the symptoms and co-infections associated with Lyme disease.

Wireweed shows antifungal properties to skin infections against *Candida albicans* and *Aspergillus niger* and has wound-healing abilities.

Buhner[64] recommends taking wireweed when there is a buzzing sensation in the body or "electric feeling" or crawling sensation in nerves. He also uses it for sore gums, toothache, and eye infections.

Observation: I have noticed that *Chlamydia trachomatis* infection and pneumonia are considered co-infections in some protocols and have been present in a number of my clients, even after antibiotic treatment. Not only is there a suggestion by doctors that chlamydia can live in your gut and reinfection can occur after treatment, there also appears to be a symbiotic relationship between Borrelia and chlamydia biofilms to survive, which may further explain the use of this herb in treating mycoplasma. Buhner[65] uses wireweed as a biofilm breaker.[66]

Cultivation

Wireweed grows in the tropics and subtropics.

How to use

Juice: Made of the fresh leaves, can be applied to skin.

Tincture: 1:5 strength, 20–40 drops, three to four times a day; or 30 drops, twice a day; use for a maximum of 60 days. For babesiosis-related anaemia, 2.5 ml, three to six times a day.[67]

Caution/contraindications

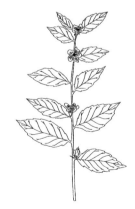

Wireweed can cause loose bowels or tiredness. It does contain some ephedrine, which is an amphetamine-like stimulant, which can cause an increase in blood pressure and heart rate and should therefore not be used in large quantities or if taking a medication similar to yet much weaker than ephedrine. Do not use if pregnant, or are taking monoamine oxidase inhibitors, or have high blood pressure.[68]

As wireweed contain stimulating alkaloids, it should not be used if feeling restless and irritable, or if suffering from insomnia or headaches, as it can be rather stimulating; it is therefore only used over a short period of time.

Woad ✳ *Isatis tinctoria*

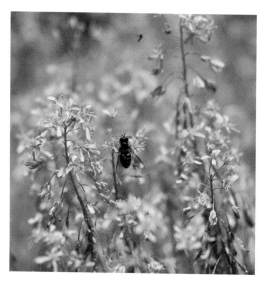

History/traditional use

Records indicate the use of woad as a beautiful blue dye for over 5,000 years. The Celts would paint their skin with it in battle to scare the enemy. This may have prolonged their life, as it would also have helped clear any infection resulting from the battle. The Chinese used it to remove heat and toxins from the blood, in particular to relieve high fevers and skin eruptions. A related species is *Isatis indigotica*.

Action: *Root:* anti-inflammatory, antimicrobial, antipyretic, antiviral.

Modern use

Today the whole plant is mainly used in the treatment of common colds, upper respiratory system infections, acute pneumonia, herpes-type viruses, typhoid fever, and bacterial dysentery.

Buhner[69] uses woad and has had success in treating Coxsackie virus, mycoplasma, and Bartonella. It can help to relieve, among others, sore throats, colds, early-stage influenza, infectious hepatitis, and mumps.

Cultivation

Woad is native to southern Russia and southern Europe. Grown from seed in early May, it is a biennial that grows 30–100 cm tall in sandy soil. It needs lots of nitrogen. It is considered an invasive species.

Harvesting/foraging

The root grows to 90–150 cm in length and is harvested in autumn.

The root is antimicrobial and antiviral and is used for acute viral infections and for chronic infections.

The antiviral effect is stronger in the leaves; harvest these in the summer.

How to use

Normally used in combination with other herbs rather than on its own. The root increases the activity of white blood cells; it is seen as more potent and is preferred for use with upper respiratory infections.

Decoction: Roots are the most antibacterial part of the plant; 1–4 g a day.

Tincture: 2/3 root, 1/3 leaf; up to 3–5 ml, three times a day, in a little water, for 3 weeks.

Caution/contraindications

No undesirable side effects were mentioned in classical Chinese texts; however, nausea has been mentioned in scientific papers.

Should be taken with caution by those with diarrhoea.

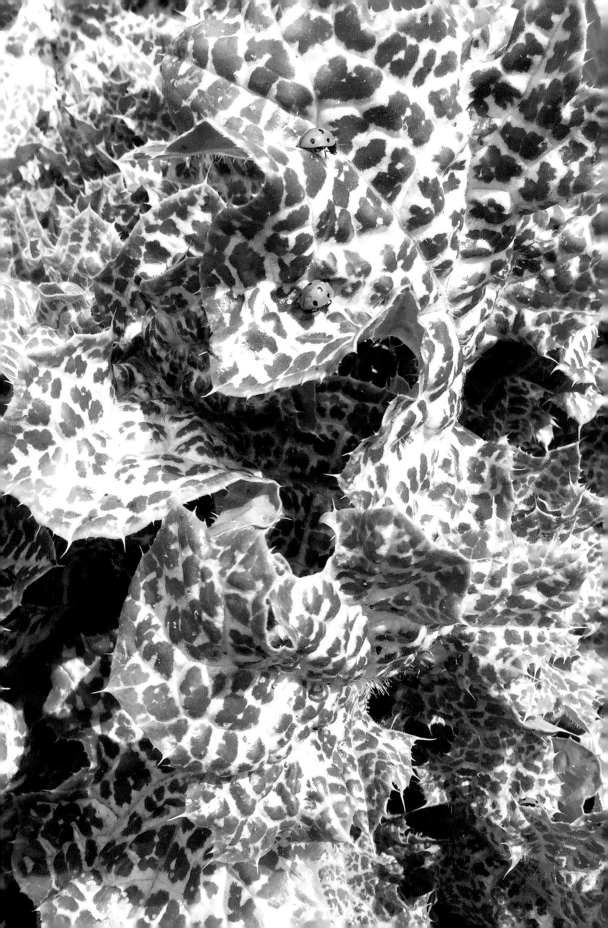

6

Co-infections of Lyme disease

Co-infections are two or more infections experienced simultaneously (see also chapters 1 and 3). When people get Lyme disease, it is quite common for the tick bite to also transmit secondary infections – bacterial, viral, fungal, parasitic – that can cause symptoms similar to those of Lyme disease.

> "I just could not get better, just constantly revolving in a cyclic round of pain and illness."

This makes it particularly confusing for the client as well as for the practitioner, who may need to be treating the person for a number of co-infections at the same time as reducing the Borrelia bacteria and symptoms. A further complication comes from the fact that many of the signs and symptoms of the co-infections may be similar to, or be masking, Lyme disease. Identifying the co-infections helps the practitioner to focus the treatment. The more exposed a person is to co-infections and other diseases, the greater the severity of the illness.

It is important for people who suspect they have been infected with Lyme disease or are experiencing symptoms of co-infections to seek medical evaluation and treatment.

According to some studies, as many as 50% of people with Lyme disease have co-infections: Babesia (32%), Bartonella (28%), Ehrlichia (15%), mycoplasma (15%).[1]

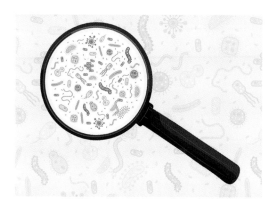

People with early Lyme disease may have a low rate of co-infections, but those with chronic Lyme disease may be suffering from more than one illness.

Many microbes can shut down part of the host's immune system in order to get the nutrients they need to survive. They use the cell signalling of cytokines (proteins that tell the immune system to do its job) to their own advantage; in so doing so, they become stealth pathogens, which avoid detection. The good news is that many herbs have a multi-purpose effect and can be incorporated in an individual's unique formula. The bad news is that co-infections are not commonly tested for by normal health care providers, only by specialist labs.

The most common secondary infections that I have found among my patients are babesiosis and bartonellosis, mycoplasma infections, and viral infections, all of which may mimic some of the symptoms of Lyme disease.

Babesiosis

Babesiosis is an infection caused by Babesia – a tiny parasite that replicates and grows in red blood cells. There are over 110 species of the protozoa Babesia, and at least 10 species infect humans. In America it is thought that over 10% of the population may be infected with Babesia. The infection can have symptoms similar to malaria, with high fever and chills. The pain in the body is often caused by the rupturing of red blood vessels. This disease can mimic and amplify Lyme disease symptoms, and so it becomes difficult to understand where one illness stops and another begins.

Transmission

Babesia is transmitted via ticks on cattle, rodents, and deer, and can pass to humans if they are bitten by an infected tick. It is often transmitted along with Lyme disease. Whether it is because of the increase in deer numbers or in outdoor activity, a number of areas in the United States

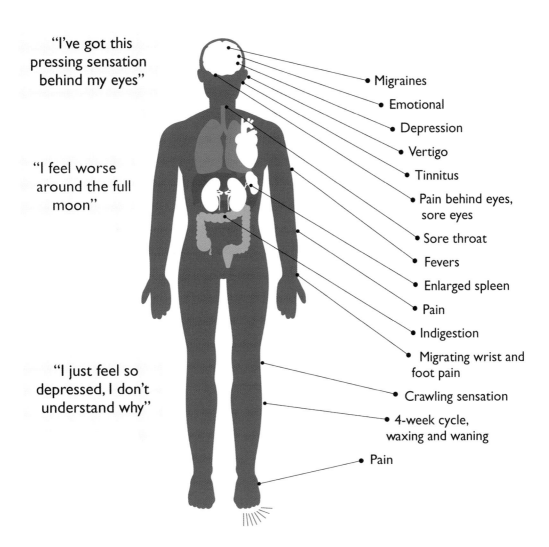

"I've got this pressing sensation behind my eyes"

"I feel worse around the full moon"

"I just feel so depressed, I don't understand why"

- Migraines
- Emotional
- Depression
- Vertigo
- Tinnitus
- Pain behind eyes, sore eyes
- Sore throat
- Fevers
- Enlarged spleen
- Pain
- Indigestion
- Migrating wrist and foot pain
- Crawling sensation
- 4-week cycle, waxing and waning
- Pain

HERBS

- Cinchona bark
- Sweet wormwood
- Red sage
- Wireweed

- Ghanaian quinine
- Milk thistle seed
- Bidens
- Bilberry

- Cleavers
- Poke root
- Ashwagandha

Challenges we face

- Organ protection
- Antiparasitic herbs
- Immune support

BODY MAP 6.1   Symptoms of babesiosis, principal helpful herbs, and the challenges faced.

are finding an increase in Babesia infection. If bitten by an infected tick, the protozoa spread into the blood of a human host and infect red blood cells. Babesiosis can also be passed on via blood transfusions and from mother to foetus. As the protozoa reproduce in the body, they may change shape; even a small change, with a slightly different protein structure on the exterior, will make it difficult for the immune system to pick it up. The parasite also keeps nitric oxide in the body low. Nitric oxide is important for cell signalling, and by keeping it low the parasite is protecting itself from an immune response. (See red sage, below.)

Symptoms

Most symptoms of babesiosis resemble those of a viral-type flu. It can have a wide range of symptoms, ranging from moderate to severe fever, with temperature reaching 40.5°C, cough, sore throat, runny nose, aches and pains, crawling sensation in skin, chills, headaches, swollen lymph glands, splenomegaly, hepatomegaly, jaundice from red blood cell destruction, sharp shooting pain around eyes and body, eye pressure with sudden vision loss, vertigo, insomnia, arthralgia, heart palpitations, air hunger, nausea, vomiting, loss of appetite, anorexia, abdominal pain, fatigue, tinnitus, mood disturbances, depression, anxiety, short-term memory loss, occasional red spots, and so forth.

Symptoms can vary, lasting for weeks or even months. They can be cyclic: some of my clients experience worsening of symptoms around the full moon, and this can last for 3–4 days. The elderly or immune-compromised are often worst affected: for those with weakened immune systems or serious health conditions the symptoms can be life-threatening; other people may remain asymptomatic, and their illness can be self-limiting.[2]

Diagnosis

As the symptoms are not specific and can vary, diagnosis of babesiosis can be very difficult. If Babesia infection is suspected, a positive diagnosis can be confirmed with a lab test that analyses a blood smear under a fluorescence microscope, as the parasites are visible within red blood cells. However, they can be difficult to detect early in the illness, as the infection rate of red blood cells can be less than 1%, but still cause symptoms.

Tests

Babesia ELISpot: ELISpot looks for Babesia antibodies. Both IgG and IgM antibodies of Babesia may show a positive result even after treatment and once there are no longer any symptoms; this can last for a month to a year. There is a of lack of availability of the test, which may explain the low statistics of detection.

PCR (polymerase chain reaction): PCR analysis can be used to detect Babesia DNA in blood samples where babesiosis is suspected. Again, there is limited availability of this test.

Ferritin levels

Babesia destroys food cells, causing low ferritin levels, which may lead to haemolytic anaemia which can cause jaundice and dark urine. High liver enzymes may also support a picture of Babesia. Complications can include unstable blood pressure and blood clots affecting internal organs.

Treatment

The usual approach for doctors versed in Lyme is to prescribe a combination of antimalarial drugs such as atovaquone (Mepron) and azithromycin (or a similar macrolide antibiotic), or, alternatively, a combination of clindamycin and quinine for 2–8 weeks.

Antiparasitic herbs

Antimicrobial herbs can be taken for 60 days and reintroduced again if needed.

Ashwagandha (*Withania somnifera*): Ashwagandha is an immune modulator but is also high in iron, making it beneficial to oxygen transport and symptoms of fatigue from anaemia.

Beggar's tick (*Bidens pilosa*): Bidens protects mucous membranes, red blood cells, and the liver cells and acts as immunomodulator. A ½-tsp dose has been used for conditions such as malaria and for cardiac, arthritic, respiratory, and urinary infections.

Bilberry (*Vaccinium myrtillus*): Known as blueberry in Europe, these berries are high in anthocyanin phenols, which have higher antioxidant properties than other berries. They help to strengthen capillaries around the eye and reduce inflammation.

Cleavers (*Galium aparine*): Cleavers have been traditionally used as a blood cleanser and to drain the lymphatic system. A very effective juice can be made from the fresh plant with a juicing machine; it can be preserved in glycerol at 50% volume, or drunk fresh.

Ghanaian quinine (*Cryptolepis sanguinolenta*): Ghanaian quinine is used in Africa to treat malaria. Its antimicrobial, vasodilation, and antithrombotic activity can be helpful in treating Babesia symptoms and to combat air hunger.

Milk thistle (*Silybum marianum/Carduus marianus*): Milk thistle seed can be used to support and protect and aid detoxification and regeneration of the liver. The seed in an alcoholic preparation has also been shown to have anti-Babesial effect.

Red sage (*Salvia miltiorrhiza*): Red sage has antimicrobial properties against Babesia and Ehrlichia. It also has neuroprotective properties, and it improves microcirculation by up-regulating nitric oxide synthesis and stimulating the endothelial cells to make nitric oxide, dilating the blood vessels. This benefits and protects the spleen, heart, and liver, improves gastric mucosa, and helps to reduce pain.

Rhodiola (*Rhodiola rosea*): Adaptogen tonic: increases concentration, reducing fatigue, mitochondrial dysfunction, depression, infections, nervous exhaustion, and recovery from debilitating illness. It is similar to Siberian ginseng but more stimulating.

Siberian ginseng (*Eleutherococcus senticosus*): Siberian ginseng helps the body to adapt to stress. Basically, adaptogens reduce the adrenaline and cortisol rush caused by stress and return them to baseline more quickly, thus reducing the effects of these chemicals on our blood pressure, nerves, etc. The adaptogens are great for day-to-day use in our modern stressful lives, but they can also help those with long-term illnesses.

Wireweed (*Sida acuta*): This plant has a broad-spectrum antipathogenic activity. It is particularly useful in protecting red blood cells and has been used in a low dose by people with babesiosis, bartonellosis, and mycoplasma infections (although it may be too stimulating for some).

Wormwood, sweet (*Artemisia annua*), **African** (*A. afra*): Artemisia can be effective against Lyme disease and co-infections like Babesia, Ehrlichia, Bartonella, and mycoplasma. *A. afra* is traditionally used in Africa to treat malaria and has a broad-spectrum antiparasitic activity.

Nutrients

L-arginine: An amino acid necessary for nitric oxide production. Nitric oxide is important for mitochondrial function, wound healing, development of T cells and immunity, and cell communication. It has a blood-pressure-lowering effect, helping to regulate circulation and protecting the endothelia cells from Babesia infection. It is found in meat, dairy, sesame seeds, spirulina, sea vegetables, and fish. (Supplements: 2,000 mg, three times a day.)

B2 Riboflavin: Important for energy production and breaking down fats, carbohydrates, and protein, riboflavin may also help prevent migraines. Sources of riboflavin include milk, eggs, mushrooms and yoghurt. (Supplements: 100–400 mg a day.)

Notes for practitioners only

Poke root (*Phytolacca*): Poke root is a North American herb that helps to detox the lymphatic system. It stimulates the production of B and T immune cells. This herb is active as an anti-inflammatory, anti-viral, and antibacterial agent. Only practitioners can prescribe and use this herb.

Cinchona (*Cinchona pubescens*) **bark** (**Jesuit bark, Peruvian bark**): The quinine extract found in cinchona bark has been shown to be useful in the treatment of malarial parasites, fevers, and nocturnal leg cramps. Carbonated tonics are flavoured with a 0.03% low dose of quinine. (Dose: 1.5 g a day for 7 days, or 1,000 mg twice a day for no more than 1 month.[3])

Bartonellosis

There are over 30 species of Bartonella bacteria. Bartonellosis is an infectious bacterial disease that affects the vascular system, invading the endothelial cells and attaching to the lining of the blood vessels of the circulatory system. It is haemoglobin-hungry, affecting blood cells that carry oxygen and causing hypoxia. It is often known as "cat scratch disease" due to people catching Bartonella from cats and the skin-scratch markings that can randomly appear.

Transmission

Transmission is via fleas, lice, or a scratch or bite from an infected animal, such as a cat, a dog, or a horse. It is commonly believed that Bartonella can also be transmitted by a tick bite, although there is no direct evidence for this; it is, nevertheless, a frequent co-infection of Lyme disease.[4]

Symptoms

Recurring intermittent symptoms usually arise 5–14 days after infection.

Symptoms can include markings on the skin, swollen lymph nodes, occasional fever, fatigue, headaches, gastritis or conjunctivitis, and brain fog. Shortness of breath is common, with significant abnormal sleep disruption. Pain can be severe and can affect individual lymph nodes and joints. There can be a burning and/or numb sensation at the bottoms of the feet – which can be mistaken for plantar fasciitis. Cardiovascular signs can contribute to illnesses affecting the heart.

Stretch-mark-like symptoms can appear on the body where the Bartonella has triggered more blood vessels to grow.

Diagnosis

Physical examination and lab test can confirm a positive diagnosis. IgG antibodies may confirm recent or past exposure to the bacteria, but it is important to be aware that the bacteria are very small and low in number

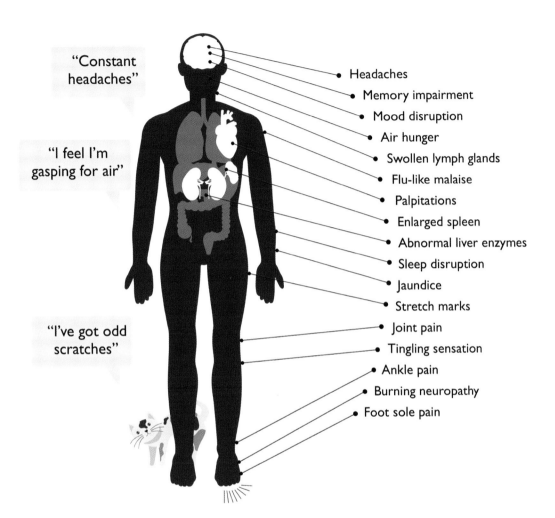

"Constant headaches"

"I feel I'm gasping for air"

"I've got odd scratches"

- Headaches
- Memory impairment
- Mood disruption
- Air hunger
- Swollen lymph glands
- Flu-like malaise
- Palpitations
- Enlarged spleen
- Abnormal liver enzymes
- Sleep disruption
- Jaundice
- Stretch marks
- Joint pain
- Tingling sensation
- Ankle pain
- Burning neuropathy
- Foot sole pain

HERBS

Reducing inflammation
- Chinese skullcap
- Houttuynia
- Japanese knotweed
- Red sage
- Turmeric

Protecting organs particularly the heart
- Hawthorn tincture
- Milk thistle seed
- Motherwort
- Red sage

Antimicrobial and immune support
- Cordyceps
- Ghanaian quinine
- Houttuynia
- Japanese knotweed
- Olive leaf
- Wireweed
- Woad root

BODY MAP 6.2   Symptoms of bartonellosis, and principal helpful herbs.

and can evade the immune system. Also look out for mildly elevated liver enzymes. There may be stretch-mark-like markings and enlarged lymph nodes, spleen, and liver.

Test: Bartonella EliSpot+ Bartonella IgG antibodies+ Bartonella IgM antibodies.

Treatment

Pharmaceutical medical treatment can last for 3–6 weeks: doxycycline and erythromycin antibiotics are often used. However, those who are immune-compromised may need a longer treatment, while others sometimes heal spontaneously.

Herbalists are likely to use Chinese skullcap and Japanese knotweed, but both potentiate the effect of antibiotics, so it is important to consider this when taking antibiotics.

Challenges:

Challenges in the treatment of bartonellosis are reducing inflammation; protecting organs, particularly the heart; and immune enhancement using antimicrobial and immune modulators. Research is ongoing, but approaches might include:

Ghanaian quinine (*Cryptolepis sanguinolenta*):   Used in the treatment of co-infections as a systemic antibiotic.

Houttuynia (*Houttuynia cordata*, Yu Xing Cao):   A fairly good broad-spectrum antiviral and antibacterial herb that lowers the specific cytokine cascades, thereby lowering inflammation and flu-type symptoms. (30 drops or ½ tsp twice day, slowly increasing the dose, or adding to main tincture.)

Wireweed (*Sida acuta*):   Hepatoprotective, antioxidant, with antimicrobial properties against Babesia, Bartonella, and mycoplasma. (¼ tsp three times a day, for 30 days.[5])

Other beneficial herbs and fungi

Milk thistle (*Silybum marianum/Carduus marianus*) seed: Components of the milk thistle have an antimicrobial, detoxifying, anti-inflammatory, and protective effect on the liver, making it a valuable herb to use. Not only will milk thistle help eliminate the toxins from the die-off of bacteria, it will also protect the liver from the damage the bacteria might do.

Woad (*Isatis tinctoria*):   The root is used as an immune stimulant and to reduce inflammatory prostaglandins. Its antiparasitic, antiviral (Coxsackie virus), antibacterial, and antifungal properties make it useful if other co-infections are present.

Cordyceps mushrooms: Cordyceps strengthen the body's resistance to infections, such as colds and flus, weakness and fatigue, and can be used as an overall rejuvenating tonic to increase energy and oxygen to the heart.

Complications affecting the heart

Plants containing rutin, like buckwheat, will help to strengthen the capillaries and can offer cardiovascular support. Other beneficial plants are horse chestnut and butcher's broom.

Hawthorn (*Crataegus monogyna*):   Leaf and flower are antioxidant and can be a tonic for the cardiovascular system.

Khella (*Ammi visnaga*):   In Egypt, khella has traditionally been used for lung, kidney, and skin disorders. Like many discoveries, it was stumbled upon by chance by a medical technician, who in 1945 discovered it to be effective for relieving angina. The active compound in khella led to the synthesis of amiodarone, used for arrhythmias of the heart, and nifedipine, which is used for hypertension and angina. I have found it to be particularly helpful in the treatment of cardiac symptoms of Bartonella or Babesia.[6]

Motherwort (*Leonurus cardiaca*):   Reduces palpitations and other cardiac symptoms.

Olive (*Olea europaea*):   The leaf is antithrombotic and protective against oxidative damage and protective of blood cells; improves healing time in the body.

Red sage (*Salvia miltiorrhiza*):   Can provide endothelial and cardiac support.

Nutrients that might help

Epigallocatechin gallate (EGCG): Compound found in high levels in green tea. It has become very popular for its antioxidants to slow oxidation and damage to the brain. Green tea contains polyphenol antioxidants that help fight free radicals. It also contains thiamine, which helps to keep you calm and focused, by elevating dopamine levels in the brain. (Three cups a day.)

Rutin: A phytonutrient that is a powerful antioxidant used to improve circulation, reduce inflammation, and support cardiac and eye health. It is found in apple skin, capers, cherries, apricots, and buckwheat.

Quercetin: Another phytonutrient with anti-bacterial/antiviral benefits, found in onions, apples, garlic, kale, Brussels sprouts, and cabbage.

Methyl B12: Important for brain and nerve function. As many people are deficient in this vitamin, it is worth having a test to check your levels before taking a supplement.

Alpha-lipoic acid: Potent antioxidant regulating glutathione and enhancing effect of vitamin C and E. It helps to remove toxins from the body, protects the nerves, supports oxygen and immune function, and can help with blood glucose levels. A side effect could be acid reflux.

L-arginine: Amino acid that helps to widen the blood vessels, allowing more blood to flow throughout the body.

   Important note: If you have active herpes, chickenpox, or shingles, DO NOT USE L-arginine.

Top tip

Epsom bath salts: Because Bartonella needs magnesium to replicate, this leads to reduced levels of it in the body. Magnesium is seen as nature's natural tranquilliser, keeping you calm and lowering blood pressure, yet at the same time it also provides necessary energy for your adrenals (and every cell in your body). As 70% of women are deficient in magnesium, it might be worth adding these salts to your relaxing night-time routine, soothing muscle aches and pains. Other minerals, like calcium, and several trace minerals, like zinc, manganese, selenium, and iodine, further provide a restorative effect in the body while flushing out toxins. (2 handfuls in the bath, soak for 15 minutes, up to three times a week.)

> "I was suffering from extreme fatigue, night sweats, heart arrhythmias and poor concentration. Her initial consultation was very thorough, which was reassuring. I was given herbal medication to take three times a day. Within less than a week my night sweats had stopped, within a month or so my other symptoms had either stopped or were improving considerably. I have now been taking my herbal medication for 1 year. I have lost 1.5 stone, I go running and cycling, my mood is great and I am thoroughly enjoying life."

Mycoplasma infection

The mycoplasma bacterium does not have a cell wall: it sits in huge numbers, creating a complex community, acting like a film or cloaking device on other cells, altering cell or gene function. This has been associated with many chronic health problems. There are over 23 strains of mycoplasmas that can affect humans; most are asymptomatic. *Mycoplasma pneumoniae* and *M. fermentans* are found in up to 70% of people with Lyme disease. The number of diseases associated with mycoplasmas is expanding. One of the problems with mycoplasma species is that the biofilm they create is capable of protecting Borrelia from being picked up by the immune system. This can affect treatment, be an underlying factor of chronic fatigue, and further exacerbate inflammation, making the Lyme symptoms worse.

Transmission

The *Mycoplasma pneumoniae* bacteria can be air-borne. They gravitate to tiny hair-like structures, called cilia, which move the bacteria around, causing problems like coughing, tinnitus, digestive problems in the gut, and even reproductive issues. Immune-suppressed people are at risk of being infected by these bacteria.

Symptoms

Mycoplasma pneumoniae is sometimes linked to a co-infection of Lyme disease but may not present with any respiratory symptoms. Some say there are no specific symptoms of mycoplasma infections, it just makes Lyme symptoms worse, resulting in chronic fatigue, visual impairment, joint pain, intermittent fevers, coughing, headaches, nausea, gastrointestinal problems, diarrhoea, memory loss, sleep disturbances, skin rashes, depression, irritability, congestion, night sweats, loss of concentration, muscle spasms, meningitis, chest pain, nervousness, anxiety, breathing irregularities, balance problems, light and sound sensitivity, problems with urination, congestive heart failure, blood pressure abnormalities, lymph node pain, chemical sensitivities, persistent coughing, eye pain, floaters in the eyes, and many others.

Some mycoplasma infections can share other signs with other disorders, such as oral cavity infections, chronic sinusitis, bronchitis, pneumonia. Other species have been associated with bladder infections, pelvic inflammatory disease, endocarditis, surgical related infections, rheumatoid arthritis (RA), and myalgic encephalomyelitis (ME).

Diagnosis

Test: ELISpot, ELISA, immunoblot, and PCR

M. pneumoniae can be tested for with a sputum PCR test. If IgM is normal and IgG is high in an antibody test, this would indicate a positive test result. Mycoplasma are 400 times smaller than Bartonella, so they can be difficult to detect. The IgM test on its own can indicate a false-positive if another infection is present.

If IgG antibodies are created, then the Western blot and ELISA test will have a negative result for Lyme, even in cases of full-blown Lyme disease, as it may be hidden by the mycoplasma.

Some practitioners have used the client response to a Herxheimer reaction from Byron White Formulas using A-Myco-specific formulas for mycoplasma to indicate that an infection is present: absence of a Herxheimer reaction would indicate that the mycoplasma is inactive. Alternatively, the ArminLabs checklist can be used to identify what co-infections may need testing or addressing in the clinic.

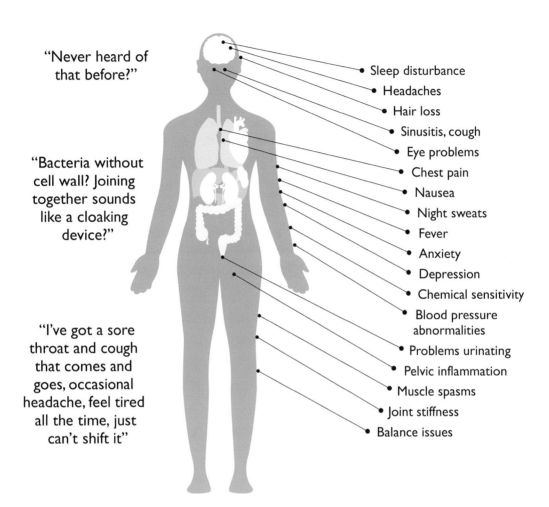

"Never heard of that before?"

"Bacteria without cell wall? Joining together sounds like a cloaking device?"

"I've got a sore throat and cough that comes and goes, occasional headache, feel tired all the time, just can't shift it"

- Sleep disturbance
- Headaches
- Hair loss
- Sinusitis, cough
- Eye problems
- Chest pain
- Nausea
- Night sweats
- Fever
- Anxiety
- Depression
- Chemical sensitivity
- Blood pressure abnormalities
- Problems urinating
- Pelvic inflammation
- Muscle spasms
- Joint stiffness
- Balance issues

HERBS

Enhance the immune system
- Andrographis
- Cat's claw
- Chinese skullcap root
- Echinacea
- Elderberry
- Houttuynia
- Motherwort
- Wireweed
- Woad

Other
- Cordyceps
- Serrapeptase
- Grape seed extract
- Pomegranate juice

Aim to:
(1) replace nutrients
(2) reduce inflammation
(3) use antibacterial herbs
(4) use immune modulators
(5) protect organs

BODY MAP 6.3   Symptoms of mycoplasma infection, principal helpful herbs, and aims.

Treatment

Most doctors wouldn't think or know about testing for mycoplasma, leading to a misdiagnosis. Antibiotics such as doxycycline and azithromycin are used as a treatment for mycoplasmas, but they can easily develop a resistance to these drugs. It is also worth bearing in mind that *Mycoplasma pneumoniae* is a common pathogen that could go away without any medical intervention.

Creating an environment the mycoplasma cannot live in is key to treatment. Antimicrobial herbs that target the inhibition of enzymes and vitamins such as folic acid, as well as the vitamins needed for cell division, can disable the bacteria so it cannot grow. Protecting organs affected by the bacteria, reducing inflammation, and supporting the nervous system and the immune system to detect the bacteria can be helpful when devising a treatment plan.

The main components of the plan would involve protecting the red blood cells and organs that are vulnerable to infection, like mucous membranes, cilia, collagen, and cartilage. The integrity and health of intestinal and mucosal barriers is associated with protection from a broad range of illnesses. The strength of these barriers is critical in stopping millions of microbes from crossing over to the host and challenging the host immune system. Thus avoiding allergens, which cause a weakening of mucus membranes, is important, while encouraging healthy bacteria to thrive, such as by taking pre- and probiotics, is equally important.

Immune system

Herbs such as Echinacea, cat's claw, and elderberry can stimulate immune function by increasing white blood cells to control microbial invasion. Mycoplasma create, cell by cell, a protective invisible mass called biofilm. This cloaking device has the effect of increasing the cells' strength in numbers and makes them resistant to attack by antibiotics. The colonisation of cells creates communities that communicate with each other (quorum sensing). Andrographis, garlic, St John's wort, ginger, sweet chestnut, Chelidonium, and ginseng have shown signs of efficacy and have been found beneficial in disrupting quorum communication.

I think it is worth mentioning that not all biofilms are harmful: in fact, Lactobacillus is a type of friendly bacteria that lives in our gut and our genital and urinary system and forms a protective biofilm and mucous barrier.

Andrographis (*Andrographis paniculata*, **Chuan Xin Lian, King of Bitters**): Anti-spirochete that enhances immune function and protects the heart. It modulates the immune system by reducing histamine release from mast cells, and it also inhibits bacteria from communicating with each other (quorum sensing) and multiplying.

Chinese skullcap (*Scutellaria baicalensis*): The root has been used to treat mycoplasma associated with respiratory, urinary, and digestive disruptions. The supplement Baicalin reduces inflammation, protects the brain, and improves DNA repair and absorption of drugs and herbs.

Cordyceps mushrooms: Used to restore immune function, support the adrenals, reduce inflammation, protect mitochondria, increase glutathione levels, and reduce oxidative stress and blood sugar levels.

Greater celandine (*Chelidonium majus*): Antifungal and antiviral and has been shown to reduce biofilm. Celandine benefits the liver and digestive system and helps to improve the eliminations of bacteria. Its pain-relieving effect can reduce discomfort in the host. Fresh tincture, taken internally, is particularly useful where eye health is involved.

Houttuynia (*Houttuynia cordata*, **Yu Xing Cao**): Stimulates the parts of the immune system that lower bacterial or virus-initiated inflammation in cellular tissue. Its broad-spectrum antibacterial effect has been shown to be successful in the treatment of *Mycoplasma pneumoniae*.

Lumbrokinase: Traditionally used in Chinese medicine. It is an enzyme produced by *Lumbricus rubellus*, a type of earthworm. It is commonly used to stop blood clotting or for breaking up biofilm by dissolving the fibrin that it consists of – presumably the way leeches were used in the past and are now for microsurgery or pain management in osteoporosis.[7]

Serrapeptase: An enzyme produced by Serratia bacteria in the intestines of silkworms. This enzyme breaks down protein, which dissolves the cocoon it comes from, allowing the moth/silkworm to emerge. As a supplement it is effective in helping to break down the mycoplasma cell walls.

Wireweed (*Sida acuta*): Has antimicrobial properties against mycoplasma, Babesia, and Bartonella.

Woad (*Isatis tinctoria*):   Inhibits signalling pathways in certain mycoplasmas and is often helpful as an immune tonic in respiratory tract infections with asthma-type symptoms and pneumonia.

Nutrients

Mycoplasma thrive on gluten and sugar, so it is best to avoid these. They scavenge for nutrients from the host to survive, leading to a deficiency of amino acids. A good source of protein is essential: it can be found in grass-fed beef, fish, eggs, legumes, nuts, and seeds.

Vitamin A: Particularly important for retinol production for eye health and to combat deficiency caused by mycoplasma infection.

Vitamin E: Antioxidant, reducing lysing of cell membranes, so reducing mycoplasma catalase.

Grapefruit seed extract: Considered a powerful natural antibiotic. It is also commonly used for the prevention of Candida and the treatment of Lyme disease and parasites. It crosses the blood–brain barrier and breaks down the biofilm coating and cysts around the bacteria.

B Vitamins: A good B-complex supplements can help with symptoms of fatigue, neurological problems and palpitations. Also found in dark-green leafy veg, wheat germ, eggs, whole grain rice, peas, beans, lentils, nuts, asparagus, and avocados.

NAC (N-acetylcysteine):   Helpful to thin and loosen thick mucus in individuals with cystic fibrosis or chronic obstructive pulmonary disease. It is considered a useful supplement in reducing inflammation, collagen breakdown, and biofilm production. As NAC is a precursor for the antioxidant glutathione, it may have a neuroprotective effect and help with detoxification, so reducing brain fog.[8]

L-arginine: An amino acid used to support collagen production and protect the heart and blood vessels. L-arginine is converted in the body into a chemical called nitric oxide, which causes blood vessels to relax, stimulates the thymus, and promotes lymphocyte production. L-arginine is found in sesame seeds, spirulina, sea vegetables, cultured dairy products, and eggs. (5,000 mg daily in divided doses.)

Herbs and foods high in nitrates (which are converted to nitric oxide), such as beetroot, garlic, nettles, dark chocolate, and pomegranate, can further support immune function by effective cell signalling and activating white blood cells.

* * *

The following is a suitable tincture combination to support treatment of an individual with mycoplasma infection while reducing other co-infections.

Tincture combination:

20 ml *Chinese skullcap root*

20 ml *woad root*

20 ml *houttuynia*

20 ml *wireweed*

20 ml *cordyceps fruiting body*

- (Makes 100 ml of tincture; take 5 ml of this, three times a day.) You may notice a difference within a month.

The dose of wireweed may need to be lowered or taken separately, as it can feel a little speedy. If taken separately, start with 30 drops, three times daily, so you can adjust the dose accordingly.

Top tip

Using olive oil infused with the olive leaf can have the added benefits of antimicrobial activity and is easily added to salads or used in cooking.

Viruses

Viruses are even smaller than bacteria. It is becoming increasingly recognised that they outnumber bacteria in the gut. Like bacteria, they have a method of communication with each other (quorum sensing) by releasing chemicals. Some viruses work like an antibiotic, killing bacteria. Of greatest relevance here is the fact that during childhood most people will have been infected by one or two of the eight different kinds of herpes virus.

Chickenpox, herpes simplex, the Epstein-Barr virus (EBV), and cytomegalovirus (CMV) are among the most common viruses found in those with

Lyme disease. You may have to learn to live with them or use herbs to reduce their effect. Some symptoms of Lyme disease are misdiagnosed as EBV, and some EBV cases may also be misdiagnosed as Lyme disease, further complicating recovery.

It is interesting that both spirochete bacteria and viruses invade the epithelial barrier and that exposure to flagellin can increase virus attachment to epithelial cells.[9] This may explain why viruses can exacerbate the Lyme picture. Treatment of them is often key to improvement in my clients.

Transmission

Viruses need a host in which to multiply. They infect a cell and then use the cell materials as building blocks to reproduce. Their genetic materials are surrounded by a protein membrane. They can remain dormant in the body, and some can reappear when the body is stressed or in people with a compromised immune system. This is what happens with the cold sore virus herpes simplex, which appears and disappears throughout the lifespan.

Active viruses need energy from a host to survive. Post-viral syndrome or reactivation of a dormant virus can worsen symptoms of fatigue in Lyme disease. Reactivation of the virus is very common, and an increase in viral load may also be a contributing factor for other conditions, such as Hashimoto's disease and other autoimmune problems.

Herpes viruses like EBV or chickenpox are more common in babies and children, who normally recover well and quickly. Yet complications can occur at any age, particularly in people with weakened immune systems, causing meningitis, neuritis, or pneumonia.

Symptoms

Symptoms are often similar:

Epstein-Barr virus (EBV):   Chronic fatigue, depression, slight sore throat, swollen lymph glands, low-grade fever, joint pain, anxiety, sleep problems.

Cytomegalovirus (CMV):   Some have no signs of illness, while others may have a mild fever, flu-like symptoms, fatigue, or tender lymph nodes.

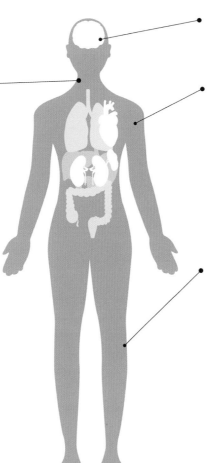

Herpes virus can cause unusual symptoms:
heart palpitations, tachycardia, bronchitis, sore throat, stomach pain, lymphatic issues, anaemia, muscle weakness, fibromyalgia, thyroid dysfunction, rashes, eyelid and facial oedema, irritability, poor concentration, headache, peripheral neuropathy, or none of the above.

Varicella zoster causes chickenpox and, later, shingles in people with weakened immune system

Common symptoms:
Fatigue
Headache
Low-grade fever
(can last days or weeks)
Chills and/or sweats
Muscle aches
Poor appetite
Enlarged lymph nodes
Sore throat

Epstein-Barr virus
Glandular fever

Symptoms:
Fever
Fatigue
Swollen lymph nodes
Tonsillitis

Associated with low levels of blood cells and platelet count, inflammatory bowel disease, herpes, MS, hepatitis, and Bell's palsy

HERBS

- Andrographis
- Chinese skullcap
- Echinacea root
- Elderberry
- Garlic

- Greater celandine
- Houttunia
- Japanese knot weed
- Lemon balm
- Liquorice

- Mushroom: reishi, shiitaki, cordyceps
- Olive leaf
- St John's Wort
- Woad root and leaf

BODY MAP 6.4: Symptoms of viral infection, and principal helpful herbs.

Herpes: Can be highly contagious and cause tingling around the mouth and common cold sores, or cause fever, swollen lymph glands, and generally feeling unwell.

Diagnosis

A blood test should pick up EBV antibodies. Cytomegalovirus IgM (Immunogoblin M) indicates a new infection, and IgG (Immunogoblin G) shows dormant antibodies. Positive result for both will indicate activation of infection.

Treatment

There are very few antiviral therapies or effective treatments available for these infections. Zovirax for cold sores is an effective antiviral to treat acute infection, but it does not rid the body of the virus.

Many herbal remedies are antiviral and affect virus replication. They should be used together with anti-inflammatory remedies and diet to protect against tissue damage. It is estimated that some 20–30% of plants from the tropics have antiviral properties.

Plants that contain alkaloids, flavonoids, coumarins, quinones, tannins, triterpenoids, and nitrogenated compounds show antiviral properties.

Herbal antiviral protocol:

> *To reduce infection:* Andrographis, reishi, liquorice, woad, Japanese knotweed, Chinese skullcap, Siberian ginseng, and fresh ginger root

> *To protect mitochondria:* Cordyceps, motherwort, rhodiola, Chinese skullcap root, Siberian ginseng, kudzu

> *To support detoxification and methylation pathways:* Spirulina, milk thistle, NAC

> *To reduce symptoms of stress:* Lemon balm, St John's wort, Siberian ginseng

Medicinal plants

Andrographis (*Andrographis paniculata*): Shows broad-spectrum antiviral, antibacterial, anti-inflammatory, and adaptogenic properties. Often used as a preventative or in the treatment of respiratory and digestive conditions, including EBV and CMV. Avoid if you have sensitive skin or digestion.

Astragalus (*Astragalus membranaceus*): Boosts the immune system by stopping bacteria or viruses from binding to cell walls. Avoid if you have late-onset Lyme. (3–5 ml, three times a day, with warm water.)

Boswellia (*Boswellia serrata*): Has shown anti-inflammatory, antirheumatic, analgesic, anticarcinogenic, cardioprotective, anti-platelet-aggregation, antibacterial, antifungal, and broad antiviral activity. This gum-like resin is showing antiviral properties against COVID–19 and herpes simplex and an inhibitory effect against the Epstein-Barr virus.

Chinese skullcap (*Scutellaria baicalensis*): Has antiviral, anti-inflammatory, antioxidant, nervine, neuroprotective, sedative, hepatoprotective, antispasmodic, and antifungal properties.

Cinchona (*Cinchona pubescens*) bark: Quinine acts as an antiviral against herpes simplex by allowing zinc into the cell, which inhibits DNA and RNA virus replication.

Echinacea (*E. angustifolia, E. purpurea*): Provides immune support and has antiviral, antifungal, and antibacterial properties.

Elderberry (*Sambucus nigra*): Used for viral infections affecting the respiratory tract. It has been shown to inhibit virus replication by stopping the virus from entering the cell. May shorten herpes outbreaks and reduce the duration of infection.

Garlic (*Allium sativum*): Has a broad-spectrum antimicrobial effect. It has historically been used as an anti-spirochete, antibacterial, antifungal, antiviral, antiseptic, diaphoretic, diuretic, and expectorant remedy and a heavy-metal chelator.

Greater celandine (*Chelidonium majus*): Antifungal and antiviral and has been shown to reduce biofilm. (Best used fresh: 10–30 drops of the tincture, twice a day.)

Houttuynia (*Houttuynia cordata*, Yu Xing Cao):   A fairly good broad-spectrum antiviral and antibacterial herb.

Japanese knotweed (*Fallopia japonica/Polygonum cuspidatum/ Reynoutria japonica*, Hu Zhang):   Used to support people with Lyme disease and co-infections. It improves the effect of antibiotics, stimulates microcirculation, has antiviral activity, reduces inflammation, and reduces autoimmune reactions.

Lemon balm (*Melissa officinalis*):   Antiviral, calms the digestive tract, has mild antidepressive properties, and is helpful with headaches, anxiety, and tension.

Liquorice (*Glycyrrhiza glabra*):   Has anti-inflammatory, antiallergy, antitussive, antiviral, anti-ulcer, and oestrogen-balancing properties. Monitor your blood pressure: it can rise during use, as liquorice increases sodium retention.

Olive (*Olea europaea*):   Leaf supports the cardiovascular system and the immune system.

Red sage (*Salvia miltiorrhiza*):   Used for cardiovascular problems and as an anti-inflammatory. Common sage is more commonly used for hot flushes and antimicrobial throat gargle.

Reishi (*Ganoderma lucidum*):   The perfect remedy if you suffer from stress. It helps to re-balance the individual, enhancing immune function, reducing allergies and inflammation, and helping energy levels and sleep. It has a history of use for treating liver and respiratory disease.

Self-heal (*Prunella vulgaris*):   High in rosmarinic acid. The immunomodulation effects of the polysaccharide make it useful for viral infections.

Shiitake mushrooms (*Lentinula edodes*, Xiang Gu):   Full of glucans and can support immune function and reduce inflammation.

Siberian ginseng (*Eleutherococcus senticosus*):   Offers mitochondrial and antiviral support, reducing fatigue. It is a herb that helps the body to adapt to stress by lowering the adrenaline and cortisol rush caused by stress. It is particularly useful for people with long-term illness.

St John's wort (*Hypericum perforatum*):   The most commonly available antiviral and antidepressant on the market and easy to grow in the garden (but it is illegal to grow it in Ireland). The problem with this plant is that it may interact with other medication, so it should not be a first choice.

Sweet wormwood (*Artemisia annua*): Antimalarial, antiparasitic, antiviral, immune-modulator, and antifungal effects. (*Artemisia annua* for EBV: 2 capsules twice a day for months.)

Thuja (*Thuja occidentalis*): Indicated where there is abnormal growth of cells, in precancerous condition, polyps, or warts, or conditions with a viral origin. Enhances immune-modulating abilities.

Woad (*Isatis tinctoria*): The root is antibacterial, and the leaf is antiviral. Needs to be dried in heat to convert chemicals into tryptanthrin and indirubin. The first inhibits prostaglandins and leukotriene and reduces inflammation. It is also an antiparasitic against malaria and other parasites, as well as antiviral (against Coxsackie virus), an immune stimulant, antifungal, and antibacterial (against staphylococcus bacteria).

Supplements

Vitamins A, C, D, methylated B12, selenium, alpha-lipoic acid and zinc. L-lysine can also be used to prevent outbreaks.

Note: Avoid food containing L-arginine, such as red meat, legumes, chocolate, and nuts, as they may encourage an outbreak.

Herbal formulas may include 2 to 5 of the following:

> herbs such as andrographis, Japanese knotweed, Thuja, rhodiola, reishi, kudzu, cordyceps
> for mitochondria support and fatigue, rhodiola, motherwort, cordyceps, kudzu

(Single tincture: ¼ tsp three times daily.)

Epstein-Barr Virus (EBV)

> herbal tincture combination of: Chinese skullcap, liquorice, woad
> tincture combination of: rhodiola, reishi, kudzu (cordyceps 2,000 mg three times daily, or tincture: ¼ tsp three times daily.)
> Do this for 60 days and see if it helps.

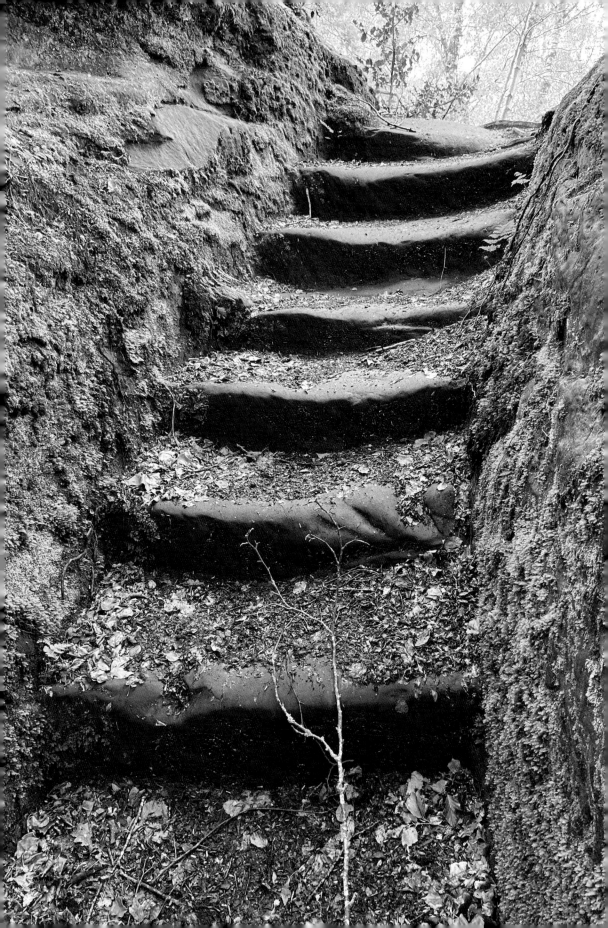

7

Self-help

STEPS in Lyme

> One step at a time – you've got what it takes.

STEPS is a holistic method I have developed to help people to understand the healing process and the connection between our internal and external landscapes. STEPS – the acronym for **S**ocial, **T**ime, **E**motional, **P**hysical, **S**elf – helps you to identify your needs, likes, dislikes, and concerns, while trying to maintain good health, positive thoughts, and strong relationships. It is designed to be a meaningful visualisation exercise to make you aware of what is going on for you and helping you to understand your strengths.

In the past, no matter where we lived, our lives were dictated by the seasons. We were more connected to nature, harvesting seasonal plants to use straight away or preserve for another time.

By becoming more aware of the beneficial plants that grow in our environment, we can, of course, still do this today. Nettles, for example, with their antihistamine properties, are at their best to harvest in spring, just in time for the hay fever season. Preserved by drying, they are helpful all year round and beneficial for the many people with Lyme disease who have a histamine intolerance.

Filling in the spaces in the STEPS diagram can help you to identify areas in your life that you are finding difficult and that you may need to work on. It is a way of mapping information to help you to see what areas in your life need support. STEPS could be seen as a medicine wheel that helps to guide the direction you are taking at a particular time in your life.

Often, if there is an area you are struggling with and you cannot move forward, other areas can help you get back on track. If you are struggling with your diet, for example, you may want to focus more on exercise and on developing emotional tools; this may eventually help you to make better food choices, easing the pressure of just focusing on your diet. If some areas in the STEPS wheel feel already in balance, then other areas might be the ones that need more attention.

STEPS: Social

The social aspects of life are of great importance to humans. We all need positive relationships, and anything that disrupts the harmony of these connections can cause stress. The relationships we have with family, friends, colleagues, and food influence our behaviour and have a huge impact on our wellbeing.

Ask yourself questions like:

 ▷ What part of your social life is causing you stress?
 ▷ What part of your life is giving you the most joy?

Task: What small changes might you make in your diet to reduce your stress or increase joy?

STEPS: Time

Time gives you the opportunity to be fully present and connected to yourself. How we manage time can affect both our physical and our mental wellbeing. Try to let go of the past and look ahead with hope rather than fear.

Ask yourself questions like:

 ▷ What is taking up your time?
 ▷ If you had more time, what would you do with it?

Task: Make time for yourself – find something you really want to do, rather than something you have to do.

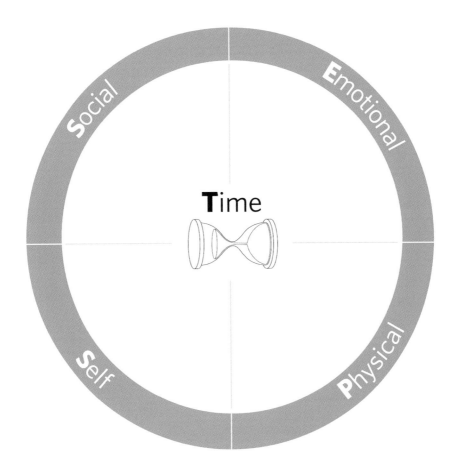

S.T.E.P.S.

S - Social pressures and stresses that affect us in our environment.

T - Time to reset and remap.

E - Emotionally, where we come from and where we are going.

P - Physically supporting the body.

S - Self authenticity.

STEPS: a holistic method for connecting between our internal and external landscapes.

STEPS: Emotional

Emotions play an important role in how you think and behave; they have a major influence on the decisions you make. Don't dismiss your emotions: they are an invitation to learn more about yourself. Anger, for example, can be seen as a tool for you to identify issues that need resolving.

Ask yourself questions like:

> ▷ Can you identify what makes you angry?
> ▷ Can you identify an emotional trigger that you are ready to work with?

Task: Is there a way of addressing a trigger, by reducing contact with whatever causes it?

STEPS: Physical

Depending on where you are on your journey, just keeping up with simple activities, like appointments, can be physically exhausting. This section invites you explore the physical tools, however small, that can strengthen and nourish your life. Being physical is defined not by others but by yourself: it can be anything from sketching to kick-boxing.

Ask yourself questions like:

> ▷ Do you think being more physical would improve your health?
> ▷ What can you do to reconnect this aspect into your life?

Task: Write down the steps you need to take to make progress happen.

STEPS: Self

Self means connecting to your inner self. You might not have a choice about your illness, but you do have a choice about how to live with it. Self is about becoming the best version of yourself that you can be. It is the spiritual element of living with illness and your shifting identity. The spiritual aspect of one's journey is individual and will mean different things to different people.

Ask yourself questions like:

> What obstacles do you see? Where do you lack support and understanding?
> Is this journey of self-discovery about recovery and self-reconstruction?

Task: Find ways to ensure you are not identified by a Lyme label.

Progress

Once you have filled in the STEPS medicine wheel, you will be able to chart your progress to your goal of wellbeing. On the outside of the wheel, put the plants, along with any foods and supplements, that are going to support you on your journey.

Introduce changes bit by bit. Remove one small thing that does not support your healing journey and introduce one thing that does. A simple step might be to think about the language you use and remove words like "could" or "should" from your vocabulary, and see what difference this makes. Above all, seek positivity, and may the medicine wheel bring you joy.

Pain

For many of my clients, Lyme disease has offered a chance to heal on different levels. Yet even when you remove whatever is causing the pain, it doesn't mean the pain will disappear.

Painkillers may have been an obvious choice for some when dealing with pain. NSAIDs (non-steroidal anti-inflammatories) may be effective, but they are not without their side effects. Painkillers work by inhibiting cyclooxygenase (COX) enzymes – COX-1 and COX-2 – that are expressed in most tissues and cause inflammation in the body in different ways. COX-1 maintains kidney function and protects the stomach lining from hydrochloric acid. NSAIDs like ibuprofen or aspirin block the COX-1, to reduce pain. Yet it should also be understood that without the COX-1 protection of the gut, there is an increased risk of bleeding and stomach ulcers, and some painkillers can also further irritate the gut lining, causing ulcerations.[1] However the addictive nature of a painkiller can make it difficult to give up, and, over time, prescription painkillers can make pain worse.[2]

The added bonus with many medicinal plants is that not only can they reduce COX-2 pathways,[3] thus reducing pain and inflammation, they also have a healing effect on the gut and boost the immune system.

If only the answers were that simple. Most, if not all, people experience different kinds of pain in their lives. Lyme patients often experience continuous pain: the bacteria can enter the joints, causing inflammation. Pain has a multidimensional root – whether it is a consequence of bacteria, environmental/social components, the timing of an event, or an emotional response. Identifying the specific root is key to healing the underlying causes and should affect your choice when selecting herbs.

> Each time you challenge where your pain is rooted, you are gaining understanding and developing an inner self-strength of awareness.

Health scares or incorrect diagnoses have led to incorrect treatment, even to surgery. Catastrophising instead of knowing can further increase the experience of pain.

The impact of trauma on our lives and the resulting stress response affects and shapes our brain. Stress activates our fight-and-flight response in preparation for danger. Constant stress can affect our immune system and increase inflammation. Short-term inflammation is, on the one hand, important to rid the body of pathogens, but long-term it can downregulate the immune system and cause chronic health problems further down the line. When people are stressed, viruses, such as cold sores, may present themselves.

Intense pain can make you feel powerless and encourage you to retreat to those places you believe you feel safe and more comfortable. The challenge is to stay motivated enough to stay positive and reduce the stressors that can feed inflammation.

"I've had a history of disastrous encounters on this very long journey with Lyme disease. This has affected my mental health more than the Lyme disease itself. As a nurse working within the health system, I will stay positive, but it is a hard fight."

The complex interaction between *Social* attitudes and expectations is the *Time* needed to reduce pain. The *Emotional* and psychological

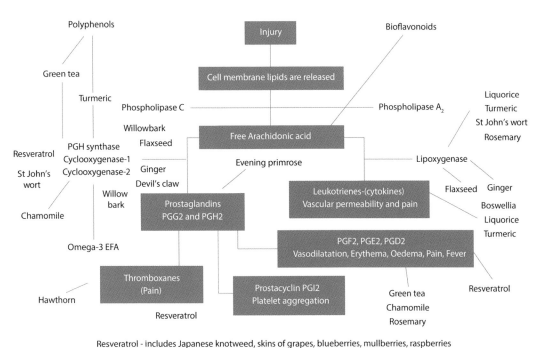

Polyphenols

Bioflavonoids

Injury

Green tea

Cell membrane lipids are released

Turmeric

Liquorice

Phospholipase C

Phospholipase A₂

Turmeric

St John's wort

Willowbark

Rosemary

Resveratrol   PGH synthase   Flaxseed

Free Arachidonic acid

Cyclooxygenase-1

Lipoxygenase

St John's   Cyclooxygenase-2   Ginger

Evening primrose

wort   Devil's claw

Leukotrienes-(cytokines)   Flaxseed   Ginger

Willow   Prostaglandins   Vascular permeability and pain   Boswellia

Chamomile   bark   PGG2 and PGH2   Liquorice

Turmeric

PGF2, PGE2, PGD2

Omega-3 EFA   Vasodilatation, Erythema, Oedema, Pain, Fever

Thromboxanes   Resveratrol

(Pain)   Prostacyclin PGI2

Hawthorn   Platelet aggregation   Green tea

Chamomile

Resveratrol   Rosemary

Resveratrol - includes Japanese knotweed, skins of grapes, blueberries, mullberries, raspberries

Herbal medicines used for inflammation.

hand we are dealt, combined with the *Physical* and the *Self-belief* system that we work in, are key to understanding the different STEPS an individual might go through. By identifying our feelings and needs, we can formulate a request for the support required to meet our individual health care needs.

Social attitudes and expectations

The difficulties around diagnosing Lyme disease can have a disastrous effect, both physically and emotionally, on those who suffer with it. Social pain can present itself in many ways: exclusion, isolation, environmental debate on a global level; it is therefore harder to get away from the suffering or media images of the perfect life in the perfect job. Social pain can have a similar effect on neuropathways, causing physical pain and inflammatory responses in the body.

Sue Carter (Director of the Kinsey Institute, Professor of Biology at Indiana University, Bloomington, and Professor Emerita at the University of Illinois) demonstrates in her work that positive social interaction is key to increasing our oxytocin messengers in the brain, and that this hormone has a positive effect in terms of bonding and of reducing stress, inflammation, and even fear.[4]

Trauma can happen in relationships that lack safety, which can contribute to patterns that come to be played out in our emotions, refashioning relationships and minds, and limiting our choices in life.

We may need to develop more compassion and understanding of ourselves, avoiding activities that can harm, and take on board healthier life-style choices. Social pressures may lead us into temptation and entice us into seeking short-term relief.

"I hate feeling so out of control with my eating, but I've got no one on my side but you."

For those of us who have addictive personalities, it can feel that parts of your body are out of control. The craving for alcohol, drugs, sugar, and so on may be the gut bacteria craving sugar for a short-term opioid and dopamine release. Temptation has been described as a gift, a warning, a red flag, and a reminder that we have a choice.

It can be connected to the deep pain of not feeling worthy and lovable, and needing to feel more valuable or good on the inside. That is why we, as herbalists, may take a holistic approach and support you on every level. To be honest, most of my clients have done a lot of work already.

For some, joining a support group can be helpful; for others, it may lead to a loss of identity. Furthermore, many people who get well move on: you don't always hear their stories, and they are no longer there to share and to give hope and direction to those seeking help.

One of the most important factors in supporting our health is bonding and forming a social connection. One of the easiest ways to do this is with food. What and where we eat plays a major role in our social lives and health. Eating food that is high in nutrient-rich in omega-3 vitamin B12 and avoiding processed food and gluten can have a huge impact on reducing inflammation. Being outdoors in the sun for 20 minutes a day or taking supplements in the winter can be enough to increase your absorption of vitamin D, improving mood, immune function, and bone and muscle function, and reducing inflammation.

Time and the reduction of pain

Pain may come and go with Lyme disease, be fleeting, move around the body. Emotional pain will take as long as it takes to work through.

Timing of drugs, monthly cycles, eating, drinking, waking and resting rhythms, and metabolism may all interplay with the effect of inflammation and pain.[5]

The time taken to rest allows us to focus on what activity it is that we really need. To remain healthy requires time, such as preparing regular meals, which could be beneficial in reducing inflammation or supporting detox. Reducing toxins externally and internally in your home, in your skin care, and in what you eat can reset the alarm system that triggers inflammation in the body.

Modern life moves fast and can create a "toxic environment" that may affect self-esteem and healing. Connections and social support can often offer creative ways to deal with stressors in a way that does not compromise the individual and may enhance proper coping strategies.

Sometimes the "work" needed here is emotional – setting boundaries or completing activities that are meaningful for the individual.

The key to a world of positive emotions may require help from meaningful social ties, from a counsellor or a psychotherapist; or it may arise from creating time and space to sit and breathe, reflecting on where the pain is coming from and what strategies will be needed to restore balance.

Emotional pain

Decisions we take and the guidance we are given can lead to a different path, and this is how we create our lives. Identifying our needs and healing old wounds through breath work, play, creativity, and so on can be cathartic.

Places of comfort will be established as we grow: a hug from your mum or a piece of chocolate could make you feel better. Yet as we

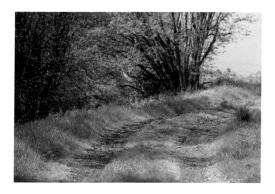

get older, unmet childhood needs and challenging experiences throughout life will no doubt affect how we feel and how our nervous system responds. Unexplored trauma may cause patterns that keep us stuck in emotional pain. We may have learnt how to seek help, talk things through, or self-soothe in different ways by becoming more resilient in the process, or we may respond to daily stresses in life by creating coping strategies.

Some strategies – such as eating well, exercise, and so forth – may have pain-relieving benefits and create joy.

> Responding with awareness
> enables you to gain power and control.

Physical pain

Inflammation in the body is one of the main causes of pain, causing tissue to swell, which presses on nerve endings. Reducing the inflammation by using antimicrobials to reduce pathogens and enhancing the immune system can help here. Relieving other "stressors" that contribute to pain will also help healing of the body.

Oxidative stress can damage cell membranes and mitochondrial membranes, which contribute to mitochondrial dysfunction in the immune cells. The mitochondrial cells contain DNA: subtle changes can cause an increase in mutation, resulting in degenerative disease and inflammation further down the chain of events. Heavy metals and environmental chemicals can also have a degenerative effect on the body.

Self-belief

First and foremost you should be compassionate with yourselves and understand that taking steps, however small, will help in controlling pain. Support your health with a personal inquiry and identify your "stress" triggers. Part of the work we provide requires identifying triggers that do not serve us, and letting go of them. This can be a personal stage for transformation, a window where synapses in the nervous system can be rewired.

Scientists discovered that a range of positive emotions, together with encouragement, lowered the impact of inflammatory processes and prompted individuals to engage with their environment and activities.[6]

Activities   What one small change can you make to reduce pain or improve your wellbeing?

- at home
- at work
- in the kitchen
- in the bedroom
- in a cupboard
- in your exercise habits
- in your spiritual/curious, brainy self

An organic diet, meditation, mindfulness, regular stretching exercises, walking, Pilates, yoga will also increase endorphin levels and improve muscle tone supporting the core of the body.

Causes of inflammation

- » physical trauma;
- » emotional stress causes cortisol to be released, lowers immunity, and increases inflammation in the body; stress can create an environment that increases inflammatory markers, affecting mood;
- » when the brain cannot cope with stress, trauma, poisons, or nutritional deficiencies, it releases pro-inflammatory markers.
- » lack of vagal tone causing poor communication between hormones, gut bacteria, and neurotransmitters; when stimulated, vagal tone can help regulate stress and keep inflammation under control;
- » fluctuating hormones – insulin, progesterone, and oestrogen – can causes low-grade inflammation in the body;
- » diet low in nutrients, omega-3 essential fatty acids;
- » a high gluten, sugar and processed diet causing inflammation;
- » allergies, whether to food or to the environment – plastic or chemicals – can cause irritation and further trigger inflammation.

Herbal treatment for pain related to Lyme disease

Physical pain

Physical pain relief can come from many other types of therapies. By choosing medicinal plants and other types of treatment, such as massage, acupuncture, or yoga, you can cover more than one base.

Green tea (*Camellia sinensis*):   A powerful antioxidant, green tea is used to reduce free radicals and inflammation in the body. It is possible that green tea can be used to treat arthritic inflammation and has cardio-vascular and neuroprotective activity. Drinking 3–4 cups a day is the usual recommendation.

Cat's claw (*Uncaria tomentosa*):   One of those great all-rounders in treating Lyme disease because of its immune-modulating effect, especially if there is an inflammatory arthritic condition affecting the joints.

Devil's claw (*Harpagophytum procumbens*):   Has been used for centuries in Africa to relieve muscle pain and arthritic-type conditions. It has also been used in combination with other types of herbs, such as turmeric and capsicum, to treat fibromyalgia, inflamed tendons, and migraines. (It should be avoided by those with a sensitive digestive system.)

Meadowsweet (*Filipendula ulmaria*):   Meadowsweet herb contains salicylic acid, which is the basis of aspirin, used widely as an analgesic. Salicylic acid inhibits mucus secretion, and without this protective secretion the stomach is more susceptible to stomach ulcers, so aspirin should not be taken regularly in high doses.

The action of using meadowsweet is similar to that of taking low-dose salicylic acid, but with the additional benefit of other phytochemicals within the plant, such as tannins, which have an astringent action, protecting the tissue as well as having a beneficial anti-inflammatory effect on the gut and joints.

Turmeric (*Curcuma longa*):   Not only does turmeric root help protect the whole body against inflammation, but using it can reduce oxidative stress, prevent cognitive damage, and reduce joint pain. Used in cooking with fats or taken as capsules with food.

Cramp bark (*Viburnum opulus/guelder rose*):   Cramp bark is used to treat cramping pain. It can be taken in a tincture as a muscle relaxant to treat migraines, period pains, or colicky-type symptoms.

Teasel (*Dipsacus sativus*):   The root has been used in Chinese medicine for treating sore and stiff joints; inulin, a fibre found in the root, may also act as a prebiotic to support gut–brain connection and reduce inflammation.

Ginger (*Zingiberis officinalis*):   Ginger, which belongs in the same family as turmeric, has been available historically since ancient times as a medicine and a spice. Peel, grate, or chop the ginger and add to cooking, or infuse in hot water and drink as a cup of tea; 3 grams a day can be added to food, biscuits, chutneys, and even desserts to relieve nausea and inflammation.

Emotional pain

Lavender (*Lavandula officinalis*):   Calming, due to its sedative action, this essential oil can be added to a bath. It is also used in massage oils to help reduce stress and tension. Lavender, often combined with passion-flower or valerian, is particularly useful for those with sleep disturbance due to pain or anxiety.

Skullcap, Virginian (*Scutellaria lateriflora*), common (*S. galericulata*):   Can be used to prevent anxiety and/or the pain that is causing depression; by working on the neurotransmitters that release serotonin, it acts like a restorative tonic.

Chamomile (*Matricaria chamomilla, M. recutita*):   An easy household anti-inflammatory remedy, chamomile can help reduce anxiety; its antispasmodic effect is useful if there is abdominal pain due to stress or medication.

Nerve pain

Lemon balm (*Melissa officinalis*):   This can be used as a tea or a tincture, or it can be added to a massage oil; it can reduce the effects of neuralgic pain, such as shingles. It can also help with emotional symptoms, calming the mind and improving digestion and cognitive function.

St John's wort *(Hypericum perforatum)*: Used in the treatment of inflammatory and viral conditions; it is particularly useful for neuralgic pain, fibromyalgia, or back pain. The herb can be taken as a tea or tincture to lift depression linked to SAD syndrome and to aid digestion. However, as stated previously, it should be used with caution as it may interact with other medication.

Pain at night

Research shows that lack of sleep can increase activation of inflammatory pathways.[7] Reduction of short-term sleep loss is an important factor when considering reducing inflammation and chronic pain.

Ashwagandha *(Withania somnifera)*: Ashwagandha is an adaptogen and can therefore act like a tonic on the adrenal glands by bringing a feeling of inner calm and acting as a sedative to help you sleep. Its effect on the immune system brings with it additional benefits.

Californian poppy *(Eschscholzia californica)*: Used as an antispasmodic and for headaches, insomnia, pain relief, anxiety, and tension.

Valerian *(Valeriana officinalis)*: Can be used for anxiety, nervousness, and for stress-related conditions such as insomnia, neck pain, headaches, muscle cramps, irritability, stomach ache, irritable bowel syndrome.

Jujube *(Zizyphus jujuba)*: Zizyphus is a cooling herb used in Chinese traditional medicine for the treatment of insomnia and anxiety; it is particularly beneficial when the insomnia is caused by hot flushes.

Passionflower *(Passiflora incarnata)*: Passionflower is used as a relaxing herb for insomnia, anxiety, tension, and pain. It has been found to improve the effectiveness of the drug L-dopa (levodopa) and reduces the passive tremor when used with L-dopa.

External use of herbs for pain: Using analgesic creams or sprays, acupuncture, chiropraxis, osteopathic treatments, and massage are also of huge benefit in reducing physical pain.

Epsom bath salts

One to two handful of Epsom bath salts in the bath relieves pain and muscle cramps, making it beneficial in the treatment of sore muscles. It is also high in magnesium, which can be absorbed through the skin.

Capsicum

A clinical study with 23 patients with post-mastectomy syndrome who applied 0.75% capsicum cream four times a day over a 4–6-week period showed significant pain relief.[8]

Capsicum relieves pain by numbing the nerve ending of pain receptors. An ointment can be made using a combination of capsicum, comfrey, and St John's wort.

3 g beeswax

9 drops of capsicum tincture, 0.05% ointment

30 ml infused comfrey

30 ml St John's wort oil

30-ml glass jar

- Heat the beeswax in the oil until melted, add the other ingredients, and pour into the jar.
- Apply to the skin to promote circulation and reduce pain sensations; useful in osteoarthritis and arthritis. Wash hands after use.

CBD oil or cream

Cannabis and CBD oil has become popular in the UK and US market as a cure-all for numerous ailments. Karin Mallion,[9] a medical herbalist, has recently written *The CBD Handbook,* which illustrates numerous clinical successes of using CBD oil to reduce the pain of stress inflammation in the joints and to improve sleep. Some clients I have swear by CBD oil, but others describe it as having no effect.

Personal motivation

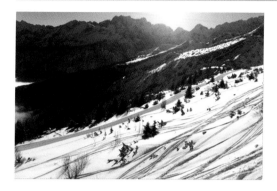

"My mother asks me at least twice a week if I have contacted 'the magic herb lady in England'!"

Identify what your needs are

"My life shrank when I got Lyme disease, I was so limited in what I could do. I would like to see greater training for GPs and awareness or warnings in high-risk areas."

Remind yourself of your improvements

Remind yourself why you are doing this, and surround yourself with positive, supportive people.

Writing follow-up sheets is really helpful in mapping your progress: how much you have improved and what areas may need work.

Choice: View decisions as active choices, not sacrifices. You are the survivor, not the victim.

Curiosity: Find things you enjoy: it may be to travel – even if it is just planning for the future with the "healthy you" in mind, embrace the journey, not just the outcome.

Break it down: There will be ups and downs. Focus on your next step. This helps break the challenge down into manageable steps.

Challenge yourself: What you could not do yesterday you may be able to do tomorrow. Step by step. I had one client who, when I asked how he was doing, said 70–80% better – he managed to rebuild his daughter's kitchen. People's expectation of what they can or cannot do or what is limited by their own body or Lyme symptoms is huge.

Manage that stress: Some stress is good. Too little, and you won't care; but too much, and you may get overwhelmed.

Some of my clients have found their family the biggest stressors in their life; limiting contact has helped their healing enormously. Others have needed me to moderate family and to set up meetings to help heal wounds. Stressor can come in the form of work or no work.

What are three things you could do right now to destress? For example, play music, burn some essential oils, breathe deeply?

Essential oils and Lyme disease

You can trace the roots of using essential oils in medicine back to prehistoric times. The Ancient Egyptians created perfumes from incense such as myrrh, and their complicated embalming methods used oils such as frankincense.

Essential oils are extracted by steam distillation or hydro-distillation of kilos of plant materials and producing essential oils in a highly concentrated final form. There are very few essential oils that can be used neat; they generally need to be diluted in a carrier.

Essential oils are not intended to replace conventional medicine but to complement it. In France, doctors and pharmacists may prescribe essential oils internally; this must be supervised by a qualified health professional and only ingested for a specific purpose. Aromatherapists use essential oils to promote wellbeing and reduce stress and physical symptoms by considering the needs of the whole person.

Essential oils can be used daily and can be enjoyed in many ways: for example, in an aromatherapy bath. Just adding 4–6 drops to the bath may encourage detoxification and relaxation and reduce tension and muscle pain.

Essential oils have been shown for decades to have antimicrobial activity, and the three oils mentioned below also have anti-borrelial activity. Not only can the reduction of stress have an impact on the lymphatic and immune system, but the antimicrobial effect of individual plants may also be key in reducing infection and improving elimination of toxins.

Microbiologists[10] conducted an interesting study on essential oils from culinary herbs and spices with the aim of seeing whether certain herbs were active against B. burgdorferi in its stationary phase – the stage when the growth of the bacteria has ceased but cells remain metabolically active.

To do this, microbiologists screened a panel of commonly used essential oils to ascertain its activities against B. burgdorferi. They found oregano, cinnamon bark, and clove buds to have the highest anti-persister activity in vitro.[11]

Oregano (*Origanum vulgare*) oil

Oregano oil has been shown to have antibacterial and antifungal properties.

In vitro carvacrol, found in oregano essential oil, has shown a high level of activity against Candida, B. burgdorferi, and biofilm colonisation by disrupting cell membranes. It would also be an oil of choice for supporting the immune system and for those who have been taking antibiotics and are therefore prone to fungal infections.

A dietary supplement is available that contains a daily dosage that provides 175 mg wild oregano blend, as well as 17.5 mg oregano oil.

Clove bud (*Syzygium aromaticum*) oil

Clove bud oil has traditionally been used in Ayurvedic medicine for treating respiratory and digestive conditions. Clove has antioxidant properties and may reduce inflammation. It is also anticoagulant and may help to increase blood flow to the tissues. A 0.1% concentration of clove bud oil has been shown to be effective against B. burgdorferi in vitro. Topically, it has been diluted and used to relieve toothache and to treat infections.

Cinnamon (*Cinnamomum zeylanicum*) bark

Extracts of cinnamon bark, from the quills or cinnamon sticks, at a 0.05% concentration, have been shown to be effective against B. burgdorferi in vitro.

Both cinnamon leaf oil and bark have been shown to have anti-inflammatory and antimicrobial activity, the bark having higher cinnamaldehyde, which has a greater antimicrobial effect.

The leaf has a higher content of phenol and a significant amount of eugenol, which makes it more effective for adding to massage oils for aches and pains.

Further studies are needed in order to determine a safe dosage for internal use.

Natural insect sprays

Deet – one of the most common active ingredients in insect sprays – is effective for some types of ticks, but it is potentially toxic. Many people, therefore, prefer natural insect sprays. Some of the most common sprays contain essential oils of citronella, thyme, lemongrass, lavender, blue gum (*Eucalyptus globulus*), oregano, geranium, and tea tree. These natural yet potent oils can help to keep insects at bay in a more pleasant way.

Natural insect spray (Kate Parker[12])

50 ml witch hazel water

20 ml lemon balm (Melissa officinalis) tincture

30 ml Artemisia absinthium tincture

Essential oils:

20 drops Tagetes minuta

40 drops Labrador tea (Ledum groenlandicum)

20 drops oregano (Origanum)

40 drops sweet scented geranium (Pelargonium graveolens)

- Spray either direct onto skin or onto clothes. Repeat during the day as needed.[13]

My client's story

I asked one of my clients, a 49-year-old interior designer, to share her story. She came to see me in April 2020.

"My experience with Lyme disease started around 10 years ago. I contracted Lyme during exercise classes outside, in the park, where there are a lot of deer. I didn't know anything about Lyme disease and the dangers it posed to human health. I was one of the unlucky ones who didn't produce a bullseye rash from the bite, so I had no idea that I had been bitten until a few years later – when it was too late.

I have never been a person who has had a lot of energy; I have always suffered with brain fog, tinnitus, and a feeling of just not functioning at my best, but when Lyme symptoms started to present themselves, it was the beginning of pain and fatigue that was to be unbearable at times. My earliest symptom was joint pain: my left big toe was in such pain that I had it x-rayed at the hospital, only to be told it's all normal – something the conventional doctors would keep saying, I'm ok, there's nothing wrong with me. The pain worked its way up my body. My back pain was the worst; other symptoms started to join in, memory loss, needing to eat 10 tsp of sugar a day to function, muscle burning, chronic fatigue, wanting to sleep for 20 hours a day, Epstein–Barr virus flare-up. Shingles would appear every 3 months. I would experience visual auras that frightened me so much that I returned to the GP. They performed an MRI scan of my brain and found white lesions. They were preparing to tell me I had MS. Thankfully, after a thorough neurological examination, they concluded it wasn't MS.

At this stage I was still unaware that I had Lyme disease. After around 4 years of my symptoms slowly creeping up and getting worse, I woke one morning and told my husband that I cannot do this any more; I just knew something was seriously wrong with me, and I needed to go to see someone privately and get checked out. He agreed.

I contacted a Functional Medical practitioner who was Lyme literate who listened and believed me. It was such a relief. I finally had a blood test that confirmed I had Chronic Neurological Lyme disease. At first, I was happy with the diagnosis, as the not knowing what was wrong with me was causing more anxiety; however, I didn't know what that meant until I started to explore what having Lyme disease really meant. I was then completely devastated.

I decided early on that I wasn't going to use antibiotics, as I had already developed a leaky gut and wanted to preserve any beneficial bowel flora I had left; so I spent a few years trying various protocols, using many different supplements, diets, and therapies to treat the disease; there would be periods where I would have some relief, but the symptoms would never fully go, and the shingles started coming more frequently.

I had to look at every aspect of my life, and I decided to move to the coast, where the sea air would be more healing. I also decided to try something new, and that's when I found Julia. In researching other people's stories with Lyme, I could see people were having great results with medical herbs, so I contacted Julia.

Working with Julia has definitely helped. I responded straight away to her herbal protocol, and I felt I had more energy, less memory issues, less joint pain. I was sleeping better and felt more positive. I still have issues, relapses and flare-ups that need working on, but I speak with Julia and we look at how to reduce the symptoms and what still needs work. Lyme disease is a moving target that I need to keep moving with. I have found herbs to be the most effective for me.

My husband has been supportive, but he doesn't really understand what it is like: he can sometimes forget and expect me to do more than I can. Chronic illness is very expensive, and he has struggled with the cost of providing me with what I need, which has caused stress and anxiety within our relationship; this produces feelings of guilt and anxiety within me, which doesn't help my healing journey. Other members of my family have struggled to understand and would rather not talk about it. I have found this all very isolating. The assumption has always been: "You look well, you must be well." It is a very lonely and isolating disease that has changed my life."

In 2017 an ELISpot testing of B. *burgdorferi* for this client showed an 11, indicating a strong positive result for Lyme disease; at the end of 2021 the ELISpot was 2, indicating a weak positive, showing huge improvement in my client's Lyme picture. The other tests indicated immune suppression with much higher opportunist infections of viral and other bacterial origin that were affecting the immune system and causing the debilitating symptoms.

Moving forward, antivirals and immune-modulating, adaptogen herbs are now key here, with focus on the chronic fatigue and joint pain, combined with therapies to support the trauma work my client was doing.

Vagal theory

"I was hoping that you could guide me down an alternative path, providing the herbal remedies I need to combat this disease, to become pain-free and restore my health."

The vagus nerve is the longest and one of the most important nerves in the body, regulating many critical aspects of human physiology. Over the years as a medical herbalist I have noticed that the vagus nerve holds some answers to supporting individuals with Lyme disease, not only in reducing depression, inflammation, and other neurological disorders, but through understanding how trauma and patterns of the past have contributed to discomfort in the body.

Poor vagal tone can resemble and mimic some of the symptoms of Lyme disease – this is why the symptoms often feel out of one's control. Stress can be one of the major causes that predates Lyme disease and the reason why people relapse into Lyme disease. When you are stressed, you release the hormone cortisol. The effect of this is to dampen down inflammation in order to deal with the danger at hand, but when the body is constantly stressed and releasing cortisol, this process does not happen. With continuous cortisol production, inflammation is increased. As the response to the immune system is not functioning appropriately, it will not recognise that the infection is reduced. This is a particular problem for people with Lyme disease.

Traumatic stress – current or in the past – also affects our ability to heal emotionally or physically by increasing inflammatory conditions, pain, and cardiac symptoms, all of which further impair the healing. The vagus nerve is responsible for regulating internal organs and triggering a relaxing response, supporting the body to heal. Its role is vital in those with Lyme disease.

Background of the vagus nerve

The vagus nerve is the tenth cranial nerve, running from the brain to the face, to the thorax, and to the abdomen. It is the/a regulating sensory and motor nerve, sending sensory information, including details about

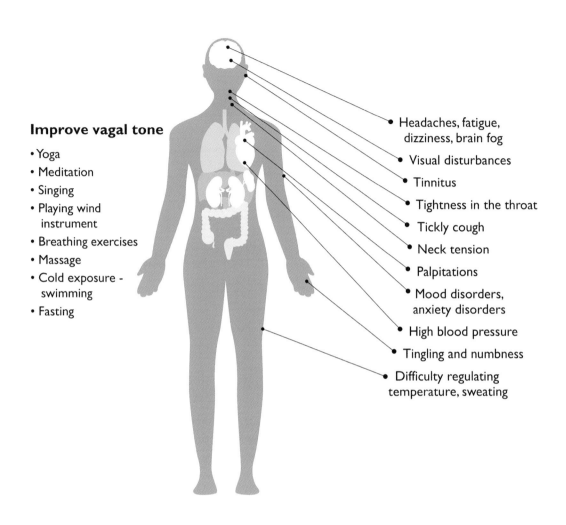

Improve vagal tone

- Yoga
- Meditation
- Singing
- Playing wind instrument
- Breathing exercises
- Massage
- Cold exposure - swimming
- Fasting

- Headaches, fatigue, dizziness, brain fog
- Visual disturbances
- Tinnitus
- Tightness in the throat
- Tickly cough
- Neck tension
- Palpitations
- Mood disorders, anxiety disorders
- High blood pressure
- Tingling and numbness
- Difficulty regulating temperature, sweating

HERBS

Stimulate the vagal nerve	Essential oils	Heart vagal	Lungs
• Bitter herbs	• Lavender	• Gingko	• Peppermint
• Fennel	• Lemon balm	• Hawthorn	• Thyme
• Gentian	• Rosemary	• Motherwort	• Wild cherry bark
• Vervain	• Sage	• Valerian	• Wild lettuce

BODY MAP 7.1   Symptoms of poor vagal tone, and principal helpful herbs.

smells, sights, tastes, and sounds, to the brain. It is the longest nerve in the autonomic nervous system, stimulating 70% of the parasympathetic fibres that control people's unconscious actions.

The autonomic nervous system regulates the involuntary processes in the body, widening and narrowing the blood vessels by regulating heart rate, breath, swallowing reflex, and digestion.

The autonomic system can be subdivided into:

> *The parasympathetic system,* which helps to maintain rest, digestion, and normal bodily functions: our rest and digest response
> *The sympathetic system,* alerting us to stressful and emergency situations: our fight-and-flight response
> *The enteric nervous system,* which governs the gastrointestinal tract.

Fight or flight

Animals – which includes humans – have needed the fight-or-flight responses to be active in defence and to survive a threat. Even to freeze is a healthy response and is part of our biological defence system to protect us. As we have evolved, the extreme hunter–gatherer responses are no longer necessary. Over time, the nervous system has adapted to the stressors of modern life. Some of these are health scares or fears of not having enough money. Family trauma can make you feel vulnerable or under threat. Adverse childhood experiences can be linked to problems later on in life, such as anxiety, depression, and digestive disorders.

Over-stimulation and adaptation to stressful situations can set a pattern of hypervigilant stress responses. This can trigger inflammatory pathways and conditions such as heart disease, digestive issues, cardiac arrhythmia, and high blood pressure. Dr Nicole LePera, a holistic psychologist, describes the freeze response as a state in which the body's response to its hostile environment is to attempt to stay safe by disconnecting from self, pain, and suffering. She also feels that "Healing is about releasing. Unlearning and breaking the subconscious thoughts and behaviours of a past self."[14]

Our vagus nerve responds to information we receive from our eyes, and ears; sound may trigger emotions of calm, fear, or excitement. This communication is carried through nerve impulses and bacteria in the gut

"If you're being told over and over again that nothing is wrong with you, but you feel there is, or that you're making up symptoms, or that it's in your head, it can lead to trauma and can be an added component of affecting one's mental health."

known as the microbiota: the gut–brain axis. The vagus nerve is extremely important, as it influences the unconscious systems within the trunk of the body. It acts like a walkie-talkie to the brain, linking the brain stem to the heart, lungs, and gut motility. Its network of branches and fibres acts like spies, picking up and responding to problems in the body that need attention. The vagus nerve also monitors blood sugar levels, blood pressure, and inflammation.

Stephen Porges, a leading figure in neuroscience and creator of the polyvagal theory,[15] explains how our bodies react to changes – in particular, how the sympathetic nervous system can respond in a fight-or-flight mode in order to defend itself, or how it can freeze or become immobilised, like a rabbit caught in headlights. Porges also explains how individuals can respond to friends as if they were enemies when the hunter–gatherer response is misread. Through stimulation of the parasympathetic nervous system it is possible to tone the activity of the vagus nerve by creating a calm state, promoting health, growth, and restoration.

Our bodily system may be responding to something, but we do not always know why or how to handle it. Our personal reactions to the world are linked to how people around us feel and our social interactions – in particular, what we see in facial expressions, whether that be smiles or frowns or neutrality. All of these influences can be linked to health, growth, and restoration. The theory proposes that positive social behaviour can inhibit the fight-or-flight response by creating an opportunity to feel safe, thus creating the vagal tone.

When we find ourselves in an unsafe environment, our mental and physical health can be affected. Our brain can misread other peoples' social cues: fearful facial expressions appear as angry ones, neutral facial expressions appear aggressive. Therefore, people become unable to regulate themselves and their emotions through others.

Activity above the diaphragm is linked to the fight-or-flight response. Activity below the diaphragm is linked to rest, digestion, and the shutting down of the body. You may find that some of the symptoms listed below cross over with symptoms of co-infections.

We can improve vagal tone through a variety of methods that reduce stress, anxiety, depression, and inflammation. Studies[16] have found that stimulation of the vagus nerve can enhance memory and reduce inflammation and the likelihood of diabetes, stroke, and cardiovascular disease. This is particularly relevant in Lyme disease, as brain fog and inflammation are often among the most common complaints.

Symptoms of vagal dysfunction

- neck tension, change in voice
- sensation of a lump or tightness in the throat, with difficulty in swallowing, lack of gag reflex
- visual disturbances
- earache, tinnitus, with no physical cause
- sensation of pressure in the chest, breathlessness, tickly cough, stuttering
- unusual heart rate: tachycardia, palpitations, high or low blood pressure, skipped pulse
- faintness, dizziness, nausea, weakness, shaking or tingling and numbness or Raynaud's-type symptoms in the hands and/or feet
- stomach pain or cramps, decrease in stomach acid production
- increase in frequency of urination
- inability to self-regulate temperature, feelings of being too hot or too cold, with occasional sweating
- brain fog, inability to form words

Improving vagal tone

When you stimulate the vagus nerve, you are telling the body to rest, digest, and even heal its symptoms. Positive relationships, laughter, massage, singing, aromatic and bitter herbs, and gargling can all stimulate the cranial nerve. Even drinking cold water can decrease the effect on the sympathetic system, which controls this nerve, allowing your parasympathetic system to kick in, thereby allowing your body and mind to rest, digest, and repair.

The fluidity of play is seen a fun mixture of the calming effect of pulsing between the parasympathetic state and the stimulating sympathetic state, strengthening positive neural circuits of connections and social engagement.

Top tips and tools to calm down the sympathetic and adrenal system

- breathing/singing
- long walks in nature, forest bathing
- minerals: potassium, magnesium, sodium
- laughter to help the body relax
- gargling tincture to stimulate the gag reflex and vagus nerve.
- massage and use of essential oils to stimulate the vagus nerve
- washing or swimming in cold water to activate cholinergic neurons, which stimulate and the parasympathetic pathways: this resetting or reframing helps slow the heart rate
- play, involving social interaction and referencing, which, in turn, helps us to move freely between a parasympathetic and sympathetic states
- exercise to stimulate fight and flight; exercising with others, providing social engagement and eye contact to keep you calm and regulate the fight-and-flight response.

The vagus nerve also stimulates oxytocin release. Oxytocin is known as the love hormone: it is associated with reducing pain in childbirth, activating labour, breast-feeding, and sexual activity. The reduction of sympathetic activity and increase in parasympathetic activity release oxytocin from the digestive tract.

Research has shown that oxytocin is released into the body to reduce inflammation and stress levels and to promote calm and positive social connection. Fittingly, the vagus nerve is now recognised and used in the treatment of depression and has been shown to reduce pain and increase wellbeing.

Oxytocin: the love hormone and seaweed connection

- positive interaction, empathy, building trust – all work to stimulate reduction in inflammation and stress, encouraging the release of oxytocin
- foods high in sulfur – garlic and the brassica family – are also important to this process; nutrients found in seaweed are high in iodine, needed for the oxytocin channels to open and be released

The mind and body

> Every time I go sea-swimming in the winter, I question my mental health. At the sea's shore on a sunrise swim, before it is even light, I hear myself saying, under my breath, things like, "What am I doing, it's too cold, I must be mad." Yet my body also craves going into the sea, and when I come out, the sense of achievement makes me feel invincible, empowered, more resilient. The rush of adrenaline and endorphins and the shock to the body can reboot my immune system, and the cold noticeably reduces the inflammation in my back. The breathing and focus on mind over matter also helps to control thoughts and to become more mindful.

The relationship between plants and the vagus nerve

The parasympathetic fibres within the vagus nerve release acetylcholine – a chemical messenger/neurotransmitter. An imbalance in this messenger can cause chronic conditions in the body as it impacts on muscle and brain function. Increasing evidence suggests that stimulation of the vagus nerve (and the acetylcholine receptors) can improve conditions such as migraines, fatigue, high blood pressure, mood and anxiety disorders, tinnitus, and Alzheimer's.

Herbs that stimulate vagal tone

Herbs to support vagal tone include those in the aromatic mint family, which activate the ACH receptors. Acetylcholine is a neurotransmitter, made in the brain, that transmits messages via the vagus nerve to stimulate the contraction and relaxation of muscles to ensure smooth running of the body and directly reduce inflammation. With age, ACH activity diminishes; therefore using herbs to stimulate or inhibit the breakdown of this neurotransmitter could be helpful. Most members of the mint family – cinnamon, turmeric, fenugreek, tulsi, liquorice, gotu cola – have been shown to increase acetylcholine (ACH) by inhibiting acetylcholinesterase (breakdown of ACH).

To increase ACH receptors

▷ Ashwagandha
▷ Ginger
▷ Ginkgo
▷ Gotu cola
▷ Reishi
▷ Rhodiola
▷ *Schisandra chinensis*

Supplements

▷ Caffeine, choline-rich food like eggs and liver
▷ Fish oils, luteolin, quercetin, magnesium

To block ACH breakdown

▷ Andrographis
▷ Bacopa
▷ Cinnamon
▷ Fenugreek
▷ Ginseng
▷ Gotu cola
▷ Liquorice
▷ Potency Wood (*Muira puama*)
▷ Red sage
▷ Tulsi (holy basil, *Ocimum sanctum*)
▷ Turmeric

Herbs to support vagal tone

Andrographis (*Andrographis paniculata* Chuan Xin Lian, King of Bitters) Invaluable for balancing vagal tone, since they work on the heart, the gut, brain, liver, and the nervous system.

Common fennel (*Foeniculum vulgare*): Calms and reduces bacteria in the gut that cause bloating,

Common vervain (*Verbena officinalis*): Stimulates digestion and serotonin via the vagus nerve.

Globe artichoke (*Cynara scolymus*):   Bitter, has a prebiotic effect, and lowers cholesterol levels.

Greater burdock (*Arctium lappa*):   Normally used for skin conditions; high in fibre and has a prebiotic effect.

Great yellow gentian (*Gentiana lutea*):   Very bitter, stimulates the liver and digestive juices.

Rosemary (*Rosmarinus officinalis*):   Anti-inflammatory and stimulates blood circulation to the brain.

Heart vagal manoeuvres

Our heart rate is often used to monitor our wellbeing. There are apps that can be used to monitor our fitness. Some herbs can improve cardiac tone by strengthening or contributing to regulating the parasympathetic nervous system. This, in turn, can have a further impact on emotional and physical health levels.

Common lime (*Tilia* x *europaea*):   Calms the nervous system, aids sleep, increases perspiration.

Ginkgo (*Ginkgo biloba*):   Enhances circulation to the brain and the release of acetylcholine.

Hawthorn (*Crataegus monogyna*):   Strengthens the heart, as it has a vasodilatory effect on blood vessels.

Motherwort (*Leonurus cardiaca*):   Reduces cardiac rhythms, palpitations, and anxiety.

Passionflower (*Passiflora incarnata*):   Can be used at night for insomnia; it is pain-reducing and anti-inflammatory.

Vervain (*Valeriana officinalis*):   Sedative effect aids sleep, yet for some can stimulate the sympathetic nerve.

Brain

The olfactory impact of essential oils has an effect on memory.

Common sage (*Salvia officinalis*): Antibacterial, is used for hot flushes, sore throats, and to enhance memory.

Lemon balm (*Melissa officinalis*): Antiviral, anti-inflammatory, improves mood, promotes calmness.

Rosemary (*Rosmarinus officinalis*): Enhances memory, is antibacterial and antioxidant.

Lungs

Various herbs have traditionally been used to support vagal tone and promote relaxation. Some individuals have found inhaling and using essential oils in aromatherapy, such as lavender, can be helpful in reducing stress and promoting a sense of calm.

Another technique that has gained popularity in recent years is HeartMath.[17] In the Lyme clinic we found several of our clients had success in managing stress and improving their overall well-being through the use of HeartMath techniques. One of the key concepts is coherent breathing and heart-focused meditation, which can help to increase vagal tone, leading to improved physiological and psychological outcomes. Regular practice of these techniques has been shown to be effective in reducing stress and improving emotional well-being.

Wild cherry (*Prunus serotina*) bark: Works by a reflex action on the gut, affecting the lungs and the vagus nerve.

Wild lettuce (*Lactuca virosa*): A mild sedative, it is antitussive for severe cough that interrupts sleep.

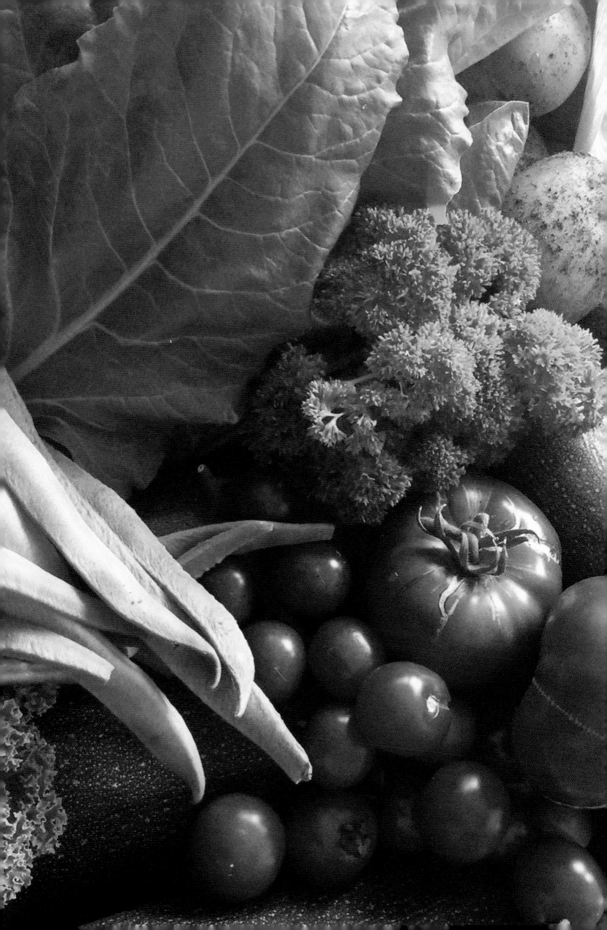

8

Food and nutrition

Eating the right foods can ease Lyme disease symptoms, boost energy, improve immunity, and alleviate chronic inflammation. But it is not enough to consider what we eat, we must also consider how it was produced. The way our food is grown greatly impacts our health. Shifting to a predominantly wholefood, plant-based diet that comes from a natural farming system, like an organic or bio-dynamic one, will provide the body with nutrient-dense food packed full of all the necessary macronutrients, vitamins, minerals, fibre, and phytonutrients to support your Lyme journey.

Avoid foods that have been refined, such as white rice, white pasta, and fruit juices, along with processed foods that contain added sugars, like soft drinks, cakes, and biscuits. Sugar suppresses the immune system, wreaks havoc on hormones, and causes major highs and lows in mood and energy. Sugar also depletes the body of key minerals and other nutrients, because it is acid-forming, causing the body to use alkaline minerals to regulate pH levels in the body. Also avoid all sweeteners – including saccharine, sucralose, acesulfame, sorbitol, and aspartame – as they significantly disrupt the gut microbiome.

Choose vegetables, fruit, and whole grains, which are packed full of beneficial fibre that slows down the absorption of the natural sugars. In addition, the essential fibre found in these foods supports the integrity of the gut wall, detoxification, and elimination.

For people with Lyme disease, it is best to avoid gluten, as it can exacerbate inflammation. There are a number of alternatives to wheat, barley, and rye, such as buckwheat, quinoa, and amaranth.

Histamine and diet

Many people with Lyme disease are allergic and reactive to a range of triggers that cause mast cells to release high levels of histamine; this is greatly aggravated when there is a lack of the enzyme diamine oxidase to break down histamine.

Certain foods contain histamine, and others cause histamine release. High-histamine foods include fermented foods, vinegar, wine, beer, cured meats, fish, shellfish, tomatoes, spinach, and dairy, especially aged cheeses. Foods that induce histamine release include strawberries, papaya, pineapple, peanuts, tomatoes, spinach, chocolate, raw egg white, citrus, and alcohol.

Some people will find that they can eat small amounts of these foods without any negative effects; too much, however, will cause a reaction. Be attentive to the foods you eat to find out what works for you.

Healthy fats

A healing diet must contain the right fats. A molecule of any fat, solid or liquid, is made up of fatty acids. All fatty acids are made up of a carbon chain to which hydrogen is attached. There are three categories of fatty acids: saturated, monounsaturated, and polyunsaturated. Different fats contain these three types of fatty acids in varying proportions. Olive oil, for example, is roughly 15% saturated, 75% monounsaturated, and 10% polyunsaturated fat.

In general, you should obtain as many of the fats in your diet as you can from whole foods. Healthy fats are found in hemp seeds, linseeds, olives, pumpkin seeds, walnuts, hazelnuts, and green leafy vegetables, such as spinach, chard, beet greens, watercress, kale, or rocket, as well as avocado and coconut.

Olive oil has potent anti-inflammatory and antioxidant properties and is an important oil to include in the diet.

Most polyunsaturated fatty acids can be synthesised by the body, with the exception of two essential fatty acids – omega-6 linoleic acid (LA) and omega-3 alpha-linolenic acid (ALA) – that must come from the diet. The balance between LA and ALA in the diet is important; the best ratio in a healthy body is 3:1. Polyunsaturated fats in the right balance protect against cognitive decline, promote heart health, decrease inflammation, and

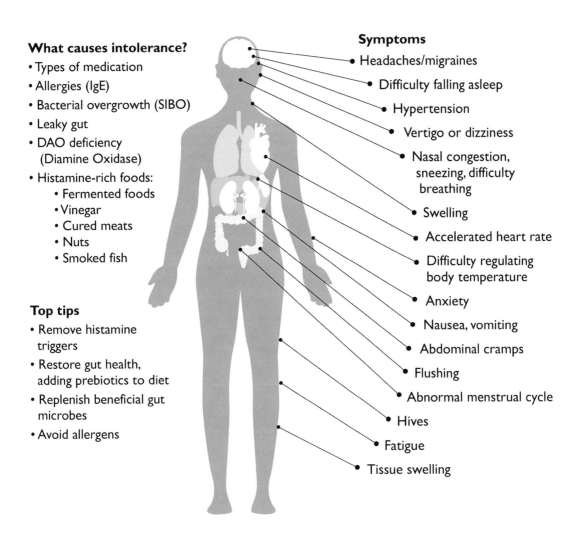

What causes intolerance?
- Types of medication
- Allergies (IgE)
- Bacterial overgrowth (SIBO)
- Leaky gut
- DAO deficiency (Diamine Oxidase)
- Histamine-rich foods:
  - Fermented foods
  - Vinegar
  - Cured meats
  - Nuts
  - Smoked fish

Top tips
- Remove histamine triggers
- Restore gut health, adding prebiotics to diet
- Replenish beneficial gut microbes
- Avoid allergens

Symptoms
- Headaches/migraines
- Difficulty falling asleep
- Hypertension
- Vertigo or dizziness
- Nasal congestion, sneezing, difficulty breathing
- Swelling
- Accelerated heart rate
- Difficulty regulating body temperature
- Anxiety
- Nausea, vomiting
- Abdominal cramps
- Flushing
- Abnormal menstrual cycle
- Hives
- Fatigue
- Tissue swelling

HERBS

Adaptogens	Antihistamines	Gut support	Anti-inflammatory
• Ashwagandha	• Albizia	• Chamomile	• Boswellia
• Liquorice	• Chinese skullcap	• Green tea	• Echinacea
• Rhodiola	• Nettle	• Slippery elm	• Turmeric

BODY MAP 8.1 Symptoms of histamine intolerance, and principal helpful herbs.

reduce joint pain. Commonly used oils, like sunflower, corn, and soybean, are all high in LA (omega-6) and are best avoided. Good sources of ALA (omega-3) include linseed oil and hemp oil. Linseed oil contains the most ALA, and hemp seed oil provides the perfect LA:ALA balance for human nutrition.

Consumption of oils that have been overheated is a major cause of free radical damage in the body. Free radicals are oxygen molecules that have lost an electron, becoming unstable and reactive. These radical oxygen molecules steal electrons from healthy molecules, thus causing damage and creating more free radicals in the process. Once an oil smokes, all the antioxidants are replaced by harmful compounds.

Saturated fats are the best ones to use for high-temperature cooking These fats are more stable when heated; unlike polyunsaturated fats, they do not oxidise and become harmful to health. Alternatively, use olive oil for cooking; to prevent it becoming too hot, mix with an equal amount of water before adding to a cool pan – do not pour water into hot oil.

Phytonutrients

The most important foods to include in any diet are a colourful rainbow of vegetables and fruit; by eating these you will optimise a range of amazing compounds known as phytonutrients. These natural plant chemicals give the colour, taste, and smell to plant foods. Essentially, they are the plant's immune system, and when we, in turn, eat the plant we harness the benefits.

Eating a plant-rich diet will provide a rich source of phytonutrients, along with an abundance of health benefits, including eye protection, maintaining a healthy immune system, and facilitating the signalling between cells. Many phytonutrients act as antioxidants – substances that prevent damage to cells from the highly reactive, unstable free radical molecules.

Each plant contains a number of different phytonutrients, and it is the combination that is so powerful in keeping us healthy. Taking an individual phytonutrient as a supplement will never be as powerful – a dish full of colourful plants is far more beneficial. Table 8.1 shows the key phytonutrients found in different coloured plants.

Table 8.1
Key phytonutrients found in differently coloured plants

Food	Phytonutrient	Property
carrots apricots butternut squash	Beta-carotene	In the body, beta-carotene converts to vitamin A, which supports the immune system and is essential for eye health
blackberries blueberries red cabbage	Anthocyanins	Powerful anti-oxidants that fight oxidative stress. Help ease anxiety and depression
strawberries cherries raspberries	Ellagic acid	Ellagic acid is one of the most potent antioxidants you can include in your diet
lemons grapefruit lime	Hesperidin	Inhibits inflammation and boosts production of detoxifying enzymes
cabbage broccoli kale	Indole–3-carbinol	Indole-3-carbinol has many health benefiits including helping to prevent cancer & maintaining good female health
cauliflower leek garlic	Quercetin	Helps control blood sugar and prevents immune cells from releasing histamines
tomatoes asparagus pink grapefruit	Lycopene	Powerful anti-oxidant. Supports heart health. Eating with a little oil increases lycopene absorption
red grapes blueberries mulberries	Resveratrol	Protects the brain and cognitive health. Resveratrol also supports cardiovascular health
spinach rocket kale	Lutein	Protects eye health, can help preserve skin health and provides support for the colon

Gut microbiota

The human gut is host to trillions of bacteria, collectively called the gut microbiota. This complex ecosystem plays a critical role in the functioning of the body and determining health. The different species of bacteria, together with their quality and quantity, is individual to you and is a reflection of your ancestry, mode of birth, whether you were breast-fed, where you've been, with whom you spend intimate time, whether or not you are interacting with soil, and, of course, the food you eat.

Certain foods are good at supporting gut health. These are probiotics, prebiotics, and fibre. For most people, including plenty of these in your diet can help ensure the gut bacteria work optimally to digest food, synthesise vitamins, promote the transmission of nerve messages to and from the brain, and keep the immune system in good working order.

Probiotic foods contain live beneficial bacteria that support the gut. While probiotics have a long list of benefits, different strains have different effects; as we are all individual, some strains may have no effect at all for some people. Probiotics are not tolerant of the heat and acid conditions of the stomach, and some may not survive in this environment. Probiotics are found in fermented foods like sauerkraut, kimchi, miso, and kefir.

Prebiotics are non-digestible complex carbohydrates that are fermented in the gut to produce energy for the host. In addition, they also promote the growth of bifidobacteria and lactobacillae in the gastro-intestinal tract. Fructans and inulin are the main prebiotics and are found in a wide variety of foods, including asparagus, Jerusalem artichokes, buckwheat, cabbage, beetroot, linseed, onions, leeks, garlic, and apples.

Herbal preparations also act as prebiotics, in particular slippery elm, marshmallow root, elecampane, liquorice, burdock, chicory root, Berberis, and other berberine-containing plants.

While some starchy foods are naturally digestion-resistant, others – such as potatoes, rice, and lentils – become more resistant to digestion when cooked, cooled, and reheated, and give greater support to beneficial gut bacteria.

Recipes for the Lyme journey

All the following recipes are gluten-free. Recipes with histamine-containing foods or histamine-releasing foods are marked [**H**] for high and [H] for low. Very histamine-intolerant people may need to omit lemon juice, which is in some of the recipes.

Gut health

The fermentation process pre-digests food, which, in turn, makes the food easier for you to digest. During this process nutrients become more bio-available, extra nutrients are formed, and toxins are removed. Fermented foods that are rich in lactic acid bacteria help support a healthy gut microbiome.

Sauerkraut [**H**]

2 kg white cabbage
3 tsp sea salt

- Shred the cabbage and place in a large metal bowl; sprinkle over the salt, and massage until the juices start to flow.
- Cover with a cloth, and leave overnight.
- The next morning place about 5 cm of cabbage into a large, clean glass jar and press down firmly, sprinkle with a little salt, and repeat until the jar is full.
- Firmly compress the layers of cabbage; leave some space at the top of the jar, because the cabbage will expand during fermentation. Weight the cabbage down with a fermentation weight or a plastic bag filled with brine and cover. Every day, push the cabbage gently down. Let the jar sit at room temperature. After a week, the cabbage has fermented sufficiently to be eaten, but you can leave it for a further 2–3 weeks before fitting a lid and storing. The longer you store it before opening, the more fermented it becomes. Experiment to find the right strength for you. Store in a cool, dry place. Once you open and start using it, keep in the fridge.

Root vegetable kimchi [**H**]

Kimchi has all the benefits of a fermented food, with the addition of powerful anti-inflammatory compounds in ginger, garlic, and chilli.

1 litre brine made with 1 litre water and 2 tbsp salt
a mixture of root vegetables (3 turnips, 3 carrots, and 3 Jerusalem artichokes would work well)
3 tbsp freshly grated ginger root
4 garlic cloves, chopped
2 chillies, chopped, whole, or with seeds removed

- Finely slice the vegetables and leave them in the brine overnight.
  - Using a blender or a mortar and pestle, b lend the spices into a paste.
  - Drain brine off vegetables (reserving the brine).
  - Taste vegetables for saltiness. You want it to taste salty, but not unpleasantly so. If they are too salty, rinse them. If you cannot taste salt, add a bit more.
  - Layer the vegetables into a jar alternating very 2 cm with the spice paste. Pack tightly, pressing down, until the brine rises.
  - If necessary, add some of the reserved brine, to ensure the vegetables are covered with liquid; weight down and ferment in a warm place for a week.

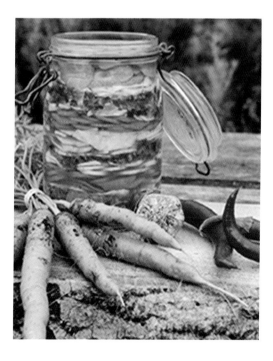

An alternative method. Grate the vegetables. Add a tablespoon salt, give a quick massage, and mix with the spice mixture. Pack into a jar, pressing down well to ensure the vegetables are covered with liquid and adding a little water if not. Weight down and ferment in a warm place for a week.

Jerusalem artichoke hummus

Jerusalem artichokes contain prebiotic fibres that pass through the digestive tract undigested and feed beneficial bacteria in the colon, helping to keep the gut healthy and fully functioning.

350 g Jerusalem artichoke
2 tbsp tahini
3 garlic cloves, crushed
juice of 2 lemons
salt and black pepper

* Peel the artichokes, if necessary, and roast in a moderately hot oven until soft.
* Pulse the cooked artichokes to a smooth consistency, add the remaining ingredients, and blend, adding water if necessary, until you have a smooth cream.

Dulse oatcakes

Sea vegetables offer one of the broadest range of minerals of all foods. Dulse has one of the highest iron and vitamin C contents of any sea vegetable. You can buy dried dulse flakes, which are very easy to use in savoury dishes. Dulse and oats both promote a healthy gut, but for some people with gluten intolerance oats can also be a problem.

225 g medium gluten-free oatmeal
¼ tsp salt
2 tbsp olive oil
150 ml boiling water
1 rounded tbsp dulse flakes

* Set the oven to 190°C/375°F/Gas 5.
* Put the oatmeal, dulse, and salt into a bowl. Boil the water, add the oil, and pour the liquid onto the oatmeal. Mix together with a knife. Divide the mixture into two, and lightly knead each piece on a board, dusted with oatmeal. Roll each piece into a circle and cut into six pieces.
* Place on a lightly oiled baking sheet, and bake for 20 minutes, or until crisp and golden.

Basmati rice and leek soup

Some starchy foods become more resistant to digestion and offer greater support to beneficial gut bacteria when cooked, cooled, and reheated – this includes the rice in the following recipe. Leeks are a good source of magnesium – the body's supply of which is significantly depleted with both Lyme disease and Bartonellosis.

(Serves 4)

> *5 large leeks, white part only, thinly sliced*
> *4 garlic cloves, crushed*
> *1 medium carrot, diced*
> *1 tbsp olive oil*
> *1 tbsp butter*
> *1 litre vegetable stock*
> *1 bay leaf*
> *3 sage leaves*
> *2 tsp chopped thyme*
> *6 tbsp cooked basmati rice*
> *salt and black pepper*

- Gently cook the leeks, garlic, and carrots in the olive oil and butter until soft.
- Tip in the stock, bring to the boil, add the herbs, and simmer gently for 20 minutes.
- Add the basmati rice, and boil for 5 minutes.
- Blitz in a processor until well blended, season to taste, and serve.

Breakfast

Sprouted buckwheat breakfast

Buckwheat – not a grain, as its name seems to suggest – contains rutin, which keeps the circulation moving and so can help to stop cold hands and feet in winter!

(Serves 1)

> *handful of sprouted buckwheat*
> *2 tsp pumpkin seeds*
> *2 tsp sunflower seeds*

2 tsp ground linseed
110 ml of your preferred milk
2 tsp maple syrup (optional)
1 apple, cored and diced
1 tbsp shelled hemp seeds

- Place the sprouted buckwheat, linseed, pumpkin, and sunflower seeds into a bowl with the maple syrup. Pour over the oat milk, and leave overnight.

- The next morning, add the apple, and serve topped with hemp seed.

Buckwheat bread

Most Lyme patients are better off avoiding gluten. Buckwheat bread is a very simple gluten-free bread to make – it makes delicious toast.

400 g hulled whole buckwheat
½ tsp salt
1 tsp dried thyme or rosemary
1 tsp honey (optional)

- Place the buckwheat into a bowl, cover with water, and leave overnight, in a cool–warm place, covered with a cloth.

- Strain off excess water, keeping the liquid, but do not rinse. Put half the buckwheat into a blender with the water and salt, and blend until very smooth; tip in the remainder, and pulse two or three times, to mix well.

- Stir in the thyme and optional honey.

- Pour into a well-oiled bread tin and leave, covered with a cloth, in a warm place, for 18 hours.

- If the loaf begins to rise more than 2.5 cm, bake before the 18 hours are up. This bread is not intended to rise, as it does not have gluten to hold it.

- Heat the oven to 220°C/425°F/Gas7, and place the loaf in the middle to bake for 10 minutes; lower the temperature to 180°C/350°F/Gas4 and continue baking for a further 30 minutes, or until well coloured and firm.

- Cool before wrapping in parchment.

Kale salad

Kale is packed full of nutrients that are critical for reinforcing a Lyme-compromised immune system.

(Serves 1, generously)

1 large bunch of kale or chard
1 tsp salt
2 tsp lemon juice
2 tbsp olive oil
1 stick of celery
1 avocado

- Wash and dry the kale/chard as necessary. Fold the leaves in half and slice away the tough stalk (save for juicing or compost). Cut into very fine ribbons. Add the salt, and massage gently until it wilts; add lemon, and massage again. Blend the celery, avocado, and olive oil together. Pour over the greens and mix gently.

Quinoa breakfast

Quinoa contains all nine essential amino acids, making it an excellent plant-based protein. It is also high in fibre and minerals such as magnesium and zinc. Zinc plays a vital role in neurotransmitter synthesis, particularly seroto-nin, which modulates mood and helps bring about feelings of wellbeing.

(Serves 4)

225 g rinsed quinoa
450 ml coconut milk
½ tsp vanilla
1 tsp cinnamon
50 g soaked walnuts
50 g soaked sunflower seeds
2 tbsp dried berries – sour cherries work really well
2 tbsp shelled hemp seeds

- Combine the quinoa, coconut milk, cinnamon, and vanilla in a medium saucepan. Bring to the boil, cover, and reduce to a very low heat. After 10 minutes stir and check the liquid; if most is absorbed, remove from the heat, leaving the lid on the pan to rest for 5 minutes to absorb any remaining milk.
- Stir in walnuts, sunflower seeds, and berries, divide between 4 dishes, and top with the hemp seeds.

Salads

Dandelion and asparagus salad with miso dressing

Asparagus contains a range of B vitamins and is an excellent source of the prebiotic fibre inulin. It is one of a handful of plant foods that contain preformed and bioavailable glutathione, a vital antioxidant that is particularly efficient at breaking down free radicals. Dandelion root is known as a "bitter tonic": the leaves can stimulate digestion and act as a diuretic, which aids detoxification. Although miso is fermented, this small amount, along with the vinegar in Meaux mustard, is unlikely to cause a problem for those who are histamine-intolerant.

(Serves 4)
  handful dandelion greens, chopped
  1 lettuce, torn into small pieces
  1 head of endive leaves, separated
  12 asparagus spears, lightly steamed
  handful sprouted sunflower seeds
  2 tbsp toasted pine kernels

Miso dressing:
  2 tsp sweet white miso
  handful chopped parsley
  1 tbsp water
  2 tbsp olive oil
  1 tsp Meaux mustard
  2 garlic cloves, finely chopped

• Place all the salad ingredients into a bowl.
• Whisk the dressing ingredients together, toss through the salad, and serve.

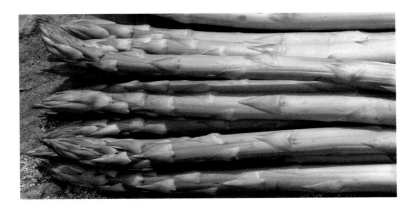

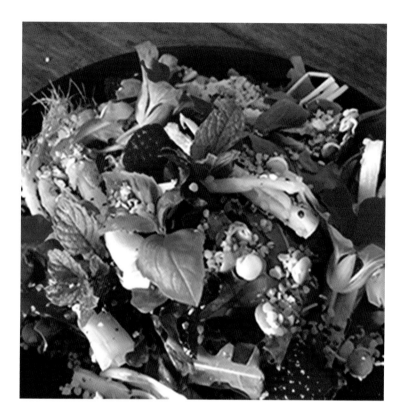

Summer salad with raspberry hemp dressing [H]

Hemp seed and oil are an excellent source of beneficial fat, providing a ratio of the two essential fatty acids – LA and ALA – in a ratio that is considered optimal for human nutrition. Hemp is one of only a few natural sources of gamma-linolenic acid (GLA), which helps to prevent inflammation in the body.

(Serves 4)

4 handfuls of summer salad leaves
2 handfuls sprouted green lentils
small handful of parsley, chopped
8 mint leaves, finely shredded
8 basil leaves, finely shredded
small handful of fennel fronds, chopped
handful of dried dulse, rinsed in cold water and chopped
8 tbsp raspberry and hemp oil dressing (see opposite)
handful of shelled hemp seed
nasturtium flowers

- Place the leaves, sprouts, herbs, and dulse into a bowl, add the dressing, and gently toss together. Divide between 4 bowls and top with hemp seeds and nasturtium flowers.

Raspberry and hemp oil dressing

> 2 tbsp raspberry apple cider vinegar (see below)
> 6 tbsp hemp oil
> 1 tsp chopped thyme
> ½ tsp sea salt
> good twist black pepper
> good pinch chilli

- Mix all the ingredients together.

Raspberry apple cider vinegar

- Fill a jar with just-picked raspberries, cover with apple cider vinegar, and leave to infuse in a cool dark place for a month. Strain and bottle.

Cauliflower and carrot salad [H]

Cauliflower is a good source of choline, an essential micronutrient known for its role in brain development, liver function, nerve function, and supporting energy levels. Cauliflower is full of beneficial fibre for digestive health and crammed full of beneficial phytonutrients.

(Serves 4)

> 1 medium cauliflower, cut into small florets
> 2 carrots, grated
> 2 shallots, finely chopped
> ¼ preserved lemon, finely diced
> large bunch parsley, chopped
> 1 tbsp lemon juice
> 1 tsp Dijon mustard
> 1 tsp honey
> 3 tbsp olive oil
> salt and black pepper

- Mix the cauliflower with the carrots, shallots, lemon, and chopped parsley.
- Blend well the lemon juice, Dijon mustard, honey, and olive oil, and season to taste.
- Pour over the salad, and mix well. Stores well in fridge for up to 2 days.

Hemp seed pesto

Make this delicious pesto with wild garlic in the spring or basil in the summer.

150 g shelled hemp seeds
2 garlic cloves, chopped
1 tsp salt
¼ tsp freshly ground black pepper
2 large handfuls of wild garlic or basil leaves
200 ml hemp oil

- Place the hemp, garlic, salt, pepper, your chosen leaves, and half the hemp oil in a blender and pulse a few times. Slowly add enough oil to mix to a soft paste. Store in a clean jar topped with a little oil for up to two weeks in the fridge.

Winter slaw

Red cabbage and Brussels sprouts are a good source of vitamin C, which supports the immune system, destroys harmful bacteria and viruses, and is needed to make collagen.

(Serves 4)

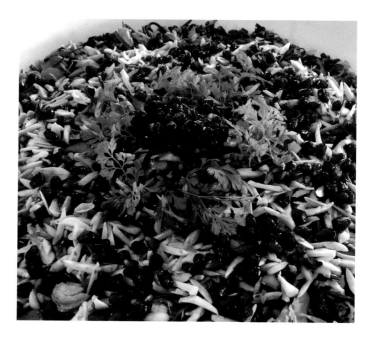

½ red cabbage, very finely shredded
250 g Brussels sprouts, very finely shredded
4 celery sticks, cut into fine slices
6 tbsp olive oil
1 tbsp lemon juice
1 tsp Dijon mustard
salt and black pepper
1 pomegranate (seeds only)
handful of almonds, sliced and toasted

- Place the red cabbage, Brussels sprouts, and celery into a bowl.
- Mix together the olive oil, lemon juice, mustard, salt, and pepper, and massage through the vegetables. Leave to stand for at least one hour, preferably three. Tip into a serving dish.
- Top with pomegranate seeds and almonds.

Pulses and vegetable dishes

Pulses are often categorised as high-histamine and so best avoided by some people. Chickpeas and lentils are high in histamine-degrading diamine oxidase (DAO), so experiment to see how you get on with the following two dishes.

Wilted greens with chickpeas, garlic, and thyme

(Serves 4)

200 g cooked chickpeas
2 tbsp coconut oil
2 red onions, thinly sliced
4 garlic cloves, thinly sliced
4 large handfuls of seasonal greens, roughly shredded
1 chilli, seeded and chopped
1 dessert spoon thyme, chopped
salt and black pepper

- Cook the onions for 2–3 minutes in the coconut oil; add the garlic, chilli, chickpeas, and thyme, and cook for a further 2–3 minutes. Add the greens and cook for a further 2 minutes, until they wilt. Season with salt, pepper.

Red lentil dahl

(Serves 4)

2 onions, diced
2 leeks, sliced
3 garlic cloves, chopped
2 tbsp coconut oil
1 tbsp freshly grated ginger
1 tsp fresh turmeric, grated
1 tsp ground cumin
200 g red lentils
500 ml vegetable stock
salt and black pepper

- Gently cook the onions, leeks, and garlic in coconut oil for 5 minutes.
- Add the ginger, turmeric, and cumin, and cook for a further 2 minutes.
- Add the lentils and stock, stir well, season with salt and pepper, and cook on a medium-low heat for 15–20 minutes, until reduced and thick.

Rosemary polenta with wilted nettles

Nettles nourish the blood, help with anaemia, and improve circulation; they are cleansing, anti-inflammatory, and a natural antihistamine.

(Serves 4)

2 onions, finely chopped
1 garlic clove, finely chopped
1 litre vegetable stock
4 sun-dried tomatoes, finely diced
1 tbsp chopped rosemary
175 g polenta
2 tbsp olive oil, and extra for oiling the tin
4 handfuls nettle tops
1 tbsp olive oil

- Make the polenta first. Gently cook the onion and garlic in the olive oil until soft, add the stock and sun-dried tomatoes and bring to the boil. Slowly, in a continuous stream, pour in the polenta, beating all the time. Cook gently for 1 minute; cool slightly, then pour into a well-oiled tin and allow to cool. At this stage you can cover the polenta and keep it in the fridge for up to 2 days. Turn out and cut into triangles. Place the triangles on an oiled baking sheet and roast in a hot oven, at 200°C/400°F/Gas 6, for about 10 minutes.

- While the polenta is in the oven, wilt the nettle tops in 1 tbsp olive oil and 2 tbsp water for about 5 minutes, until all the water has evaporated.
- Divide the nettles between four plates, and top with the polenta.

Sweet moments

Summer smoothie

The anthocyanins in blueberries help fight oxidative stress; in particular, they support the heart and circulatory system. Pomegranate juice is full of antioxidants, is antimicrobial, and acts as a mast cell stabiliser.

(Serves 2)

250 g blueberries
2 tbsp shelled hemp seeds
250 ml pomegranate juice
small knob of ginger, peeled and grated

- Blitz all ingredients together and serve.

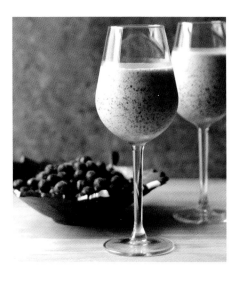

Autumn smoothie

Pears, loaded with antioxidants, are an excellent choice to help with inflammatory conditions.

(Serves 2)

> 4 fresh figs, hard tip removed
> 2 pears, quartered and cored
> 200 ml hemp milk
> 1 tsp shiitake powder

* Put all the ingredients in a blender and blend until the mixture is smooth. Pour into a glass and drink.

Hemp-chocolate energy balls [**H**]

Cacao is packed full of vitamins and minerals, including B vitamins, manganese, zinc, copper, and iron. It is also a fantastic source of the stress-busting mineral magnesium.

> 100 g walnuts, chopped
> 75 g raisins
> 1 tbsp flaxseed, ground
> 2 tbsp raw cacao
> 1 tbsp honey
> 2 tbsp almond butter
> 50 g hemp seed, shelled

* Process all the ingredients together except the hemp. Roll into balls, roll in the hemp, and chill in the fridge.

Chia pudding

Chia seeds are a good source of protein, vitamins, and minerals. They are rich in omega-3 ALA, which helps to control inflammation. Research suggests that chia seeds can help maintain normal blood sugar levels.

(Serves 1)

> 120 ml of coconut milk
> 2 tbsp chia seeds
> fruit, nuts, seeds (optional)

* Put the chia seeds into a bowl, and stir in the milk.
* Let sit for 10 minutes, then stir again.
* Refrigerate for at least an hour (or overnight, ready for breakfast)
* Serve as is, or top with fruit, nuts, and seeds.

Collagen support

Collagen is a protein that binds the whole body together, providing building blocks for structure, strength, and flexibility. Ensuring that the body has all the nutrients it needs to make collagen is vitally important during the menopause and helpful for those experiencing aching joints, weak muscles, or brittle hair and nails.

Some microbes, including Borrelia, the bacteria that causes Lyme disease, have an affinity for connective tissue and can cause significant damage by breaking down collagen.

In healthy people, collagen breakdown by microbes is probably occurring at a very low level, but the immune system prevents any significant damage, and they're able to constantly rebuild new collagen. If the immune system is compromised and microbes are allowed to flourish, collagen is broken down and not replaced.

Nutrients required to make collagen

Vitamin C: Vitamin C adds oxygen and hydrogen to amino acids, so that they can do their part in collagen production. Vitamin C is found in many fruit and vegetables, such as broccoli, citrus fruit, kale, peppers, and strawberries.

Anthocyanins: Anthocyanins have the ability to suppress inflammation and stabilise collagen by preventing free radical damage, which inhibits enzymes from clinging to collagen. Anthocyanins are found in blackberries, blueberries, red cabbage, aubergine, and cherries.

Copper: Copper increases the production of collagen and is found in lentils, almonds, apricots, raw cacao, mushrooms, and greens.

Glycine: An amino acid that is an essential part of collagen. Glycine is essential to the body's synthesis of the potent antioxidant glutathione, which protects cells from damage. Glycine is found in sesame seeds, pumpkin seeds, watercress, lentils, sea vegetables, and legumes.

Lysine: The amino acid lysine is used in making collagen and protects collagen from breakdown. It helps prevent the loss of bone mineral density, due to its ability to increase intestinal calcium absorption. It is found in nutritional yeast, sea vegetables, and spirulina.

Arginine or L-arginine: An amino acid made in the body. Studies[1] suggest that arginine stimulates collagen synthesis and makes the bone cells responsible for making new bone (osteoblasts) more active. Found in sesame seeds, spirulina, sea vegetables, cultured dairy products, and eggs.

Proline: An amino acid that helps in the formation of collagen; it is found in mushrooms, cabbage, asparagus, and kombu.

Vitamin A: Helps to stimulate the production of collagen and is only found in animal-derived foods (in its complete, active form, called retinol). Fruit and vegetables are, on the other hand, high in phytonutrients called carotenoids (precursors of vitamin A), which the body must then convert to vitamin A. Good sources of beta carotene are broccoli, carrots, kale, squash, and sweet potatoes.

Manganese: Increases production of collagen and is found in leafy vegetables, nuts, sea vegetables, and whole grains.

Zinc: Activates the proteins responsible for making collagen and is found in seeds, nuts, beans, mushrooms, and garlic.

Collagen support tonic broth

A plant-based version of bone broth.

2 strips kombu
small handful dulse
6 shallots, chopped
150 g shiitake
handful fresh parsley
2½ cm knob turmeric, roughly chopped
2½ cm knob of ginger, roughly chopped
2 beetroot, peeled and chopped
½ small red cabbage, chopped
handful kale
handful fresh coriander
1 tsp fennel seeds
4 garlic cloves, chopped
3 litre filtered water

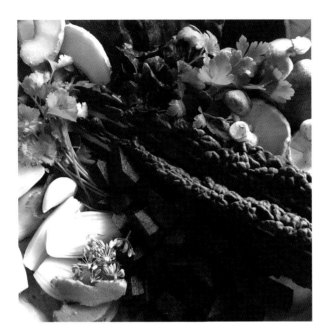

- Place all the ingredients together in a pan and leave to soak overnight.
- Bring to the boil, lower the heat, and simmer gently for half an hour.
- Strain the broth, and store in the fridge or freezer.
- Drink a cup daily, or make a soup, adding raw, vitamin-C-rich, finely chopped red pepper and watercress to the hot tonic broth.

Sugar and blood glucose

A vast amount of research shows that consuming simple sugars can take a devastating toll on your health. Eliminating, or at least severely limiting, simple sugars can help to stabilise blood glucose and improve a person's resilience to Lyme disease.

Many foods, such as fruit and vegetables, contain sugar, but they are also packed full of nutrients and fibre that benefit your health. It is the added simple sugars in drinks, sweets, cakes, biscuits, and desserts that disrupt blood glucose and contribute to so many health problems.

Two key simple sugars are *glucose*, which is the most rapidly metabolised sugar and can send your blood sugar levels skyrocketing, and *fructose*, which is metabolised by the liver. Too much fructose in the liver creates a cascade of metabolic problems that include fatty liver disease, inflammation, and weight gain.

These two sugars are found in most of our common sweeteners.

Common sweeteners

White sugar, also known as sucrose: A highly processed and refined product that comes from sugar cane or sugar beet. It consists of 50% glucose and 50% fructose.

High-fructose corn syrup: Made by converting corn starch into a sweetener; it has provided a "cheap" sugar alternative in the food processing industry. It is generally 55% fructose and 45% glucose.

Brown rice syrup: Very processed and is essentially glucose.

Agave: 90% fructose and is generally a highly processed product.

Coconut sugar: Contains inulin, which can help stabilise blood sugar, but its sucrose content is 80%.

Maple syrup: Contains 75% sucrose but also contains beneficial antioxidants and minerals.

Barley malt: A sweetener that is made out of sprouted barley. It contains 65% maltose (essentially a form of glucose), 30% complex carbohydrates, and 3% protein.

Brown sugar: White sugar with some molasses remaining in it, or added back after processing.

Honey: Made up of 40% fructose and 30% glucose, plus water. Raw honey contains beneficial flavonoid antioxidants, vitamin C, amino acids, and minerals. It has antimicrobial properties, and some research suggests it can alleviate certain allergy symptoms.

Artificial sweeteners: When these were first introduced, they seemed like good alternatives to sugar. However, these chemical, fake sweeteners are linked to weight gain, diabetes, heart disease, and a number of other health risks.

Insulin

When you eat, your blood sugar rises, which prompts your pancreas to release insulin into your bloodstream. Insulin sends a signal to your muscle cells that they need to take up the excess sugar. Your muscle cells either use up the glucose as an energy source or store it in a slightly altered form, called glycogen.

When you have not eaten for several hours, your blood sugar starts to fall. To restore equilibrium, your pancreas pumps out a complementary hormone, called glucagon, which converts the glycogen back into glucose and then sends it back into your bloodstream. If all goes well, your pancreas produces just enough of these hormones at just the right time to keep your blood glucose within optimal levels.

When your diet includes many foods high in simple sugars, this highly tuned system spirals out of control, leading to many disorders, including:

- an increased risk of insulin resistance and Type 2 diabetes
- suppression of the immune system
- gut dysbiosis, causing intestinal permeability, leading to a leaky gut
- exacerbation of anxiety and depression
- an increase in uric acid levels in the blood, increasing the risk of developing or worsening inflammatory conditions like arthritis
- an increased risk of heart disease
- risk of non-alcoholic fatty liver disease
- an increased risk of impaired memory and dementia
- an increased risk of breast cancer and metastasis to the lungs
- an upset in mineral balance, especially depleted chromium, copper, calcium, and magnesium

Often we are caught in a vicious sugar cycle, craving the feel-good factor it creates. Eating sugar activates the brain's reward circuitry, making it release dopamine – a hormone that delivers powerful feelings of satisfaction. Sugar addicts crave the repetition of the dopamine feel-good response. The high can only leads to a crash when the brain counters the dopamine with serotonin, the sleep-regulating hormone, which leads to a crash, followed by a desire for more sugar.

It requires a certain amount of willpower and support to break the habit. Key to this is eliminating stress triggers and finding better sweet options – healthy treats – as well as nutrition and herbal support.

Better sweet options

Xylitol: A sugar alcohol used as a sweetener, Xylitol came to the commercial market a number of years ago and was promoted by dentists as a preferred sugar alternative. Xylitol does not break down in the system, the way sugar does, and it can help keep a neutral pH level in the mouth, as well as preventing bacteria from sticking to the teeth.

Xylitol looks like a white granulated sugar and is slightly sweeter. Make sure you source 100% birch-tree extract, as there are other variations, including corn, on the market. Xylitol has a very low glycaemic index (GI: the speed at which the food raises the blood glucose level) of around 7, compared to 60–70 for table sugar. When consumed in excess, it can, for some people, cause bloating and diarrhoea.

Stevia: Whole-leaf stevia is sweeter than sugar but does not raise blood sugar levels, so is a healthy alternative to sugar. The plant originally came from Paraguay and Brazil, but it can be grown in Europe. It is important to note that the white over-the-counter version is highly processed and does not contain all the benefits of the raw leaf, which also has slight bitter qualities. Stevia leaf extract has been shown to exhibit antimicrobial activity against *Borrelia burgdorferi* spirochetes and is considered a natural therapy in treating Lyme disease.

Treats

Chocolate: Studies[2] show that raw dark chocolate with 80% cacao can be very beneficial for you. It is an excellent source of magnesium, and its antioxidant effect can reduce inflammation.

Dark chocolate contains an amino acid – phenylalanine – which plays a key role in dopamine production. The medicinal benefits of two pieces

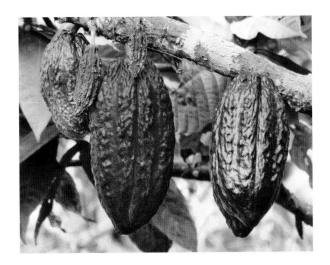

of good-quality chocolate a day could lift your mood. Other benefits come from the nitric oxide found in dark chocolate, which helps to dilate and strengthen blood vessels.

Dates: Having a few dates instead of sugary processed foods can give you a sweet fix and also provide you with healthy nutrients. Dates are a good source of fibre, potassium, iron, and beneficial plant compounds. While they are very nutritious, they are also very sweet, so you only need a couple. You could pair them with walnuts, which are a good source of beneficial omega-3 fat.

Nutrition

Eating regularly and ensuring you include good-quality protein (hemp, eggs, fish, hazelnuts, almonds, peas, beans) and fats (hemp, linseed, chia seeds, olive oil, walnuts, pumpkin seeds) can help stop sugar cravings.

Magnesium found in kelp, oats, cacao, green leaves, and seeds helps to control blood glucose.

Use plenty of garlic in your cooking: it has a beneficial effect on blood sugar.

Herbal help: Herbs with a beneficial effect on blood sugar levels include bitter melon, fenugreek, dandelion root, berberine-containing plants, and cinnamon.

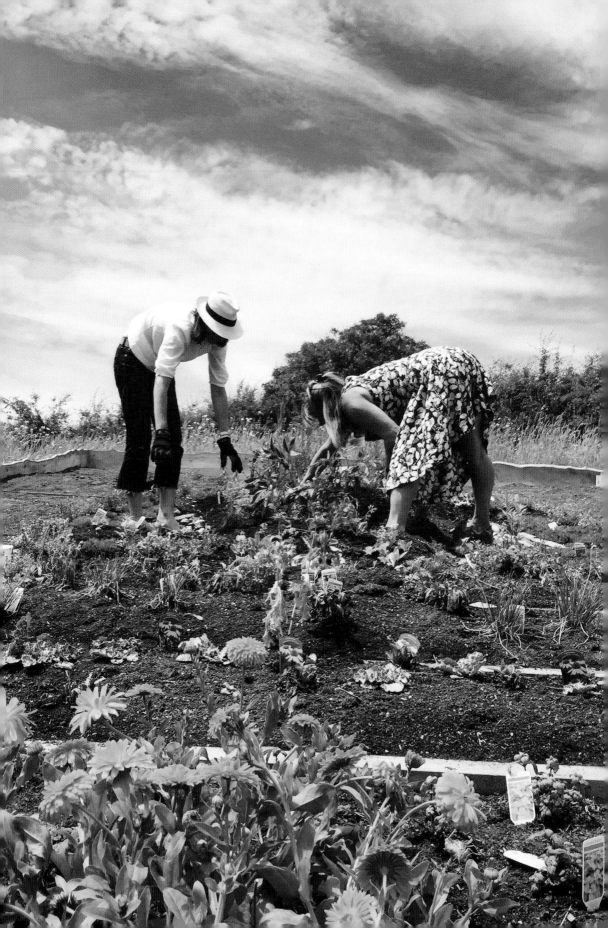

9

Grow your own herbal medicine

Plants to grow for yourself

Plants, especially herbs, have played a crucial role in our evolutionary history, with many of their medicinal properties sustaining human health. We have seen that there are many medicinal plants and trees that can be very effective in the treatment and support of people with Lyme disease.

**There are many good reasons
to grow your own medicinal plants**

» Health care begins at home: growing herbs can help create health on a daily basis.
» Our health can often feel out of our control; using herbs that you grow, to support yourself and the ones you love, provides a sense of security.
» Using medicinal plants from your own garden can help to reduce pressure on the health care system.
» Engagement in shared growing in a community garden can enhance relationships and minimise social isolation.
» Being outdoors is a natural stress reliever: it can help to reduce blood pressure, strengthen the immune system, ease depression, and improve mood.
» Growing a few herbs involves minimal effort for those who tire easily.
» Growing plants helps the environment, as well as your health: "There is nothing better than eating food or herbs that you have grown in your own garden."

Growing a few medicinal plants, be it in the garden, on a balcony or windowsill, or in a community garden, is a wonderful way to provide yourself with natural remedies.

Many medicinal plants can be pretty easy to grow, though some will only grow and flourish in a particular climate or habitat. Most will need a little sun and free-draining soil. There are a few exceptions, of course: meadowsweet likes to grow beside ponds or streams, and some mints are quite happy in semi-shade.

Herbs to grow in a container

Rosemary, mint, chamomile, and feverfew all grow especially well in a pot on a well-lit windowsill – though they will, of course, also grow well in the garden.

Camomile (*Matricaria chamomilla, Matricaria recutita*): Grows well from seed, or you can buy a plant from a nursery.

> ▹ *Parts used:* flowers.
> ▹ *Good for:* soothing the digestive and nervous system: a herb that can help with stress, sleep, and an upset digestion. It is very gentle and makes a great herbal tea.

Feverfew (*Tanacetum parthenium*): Grows well from seed; can also be grown from cuttings and division.

> ▹ *Parts used:* leaves and flowers.
> ▹ *Good for:* headaches, muscle cramps, fevers; reduces inflammation.

Lemon balm (*Melissa officinalis*): Easy to grow from cuttings, small pieces of root, or seeds; fresh or dried, it has a wonderful lemon aroma.

> ▹ *Good for:* nervous disorders, depression, anxiety, palpitations, tension headaches, and improving digestion; with the added benefit of being antiviral.

Mint: One of the easiest herbs to grow, and the plants are easy to source. You can also start a plant from a small cutting. The fragrant aroma of mint grown indoors is very uplifting.

> ▹ *Part used:* leaves.
> ▹ *Good for:* often used as a calming herb for intestinal colic, nausea, diarrhoea, the common cold, and to reduce flatulence. Can be taken fresh, or dried and used as a tea.

Rosemary (*Rosmarinus officinalis*):   Easy to buy as a plant, or you can start from a cutting. You can harvest the leaves of this aromatic evergreen all year round.

- *Part used:* leaves.
- *Good for:* poor circulation or cognitive function, fatigue, depression, migraines, headaches, flitting pain, inflammation of the gallbladder. Taken as a tea, or the essential oil is diluted into a massage oil and massaged into aching joints.

Herbs to grow in the garden

Chinese skullcap (*Scutellaria baicalensis*):   Grows best from cuttings or division, in a moderately fertile soil. Alternatively, purchase a plant from a nursery. Mulch well over winter in cold areas.

- *Part used:* roots.
- *Good for:* reducing inflammation related to allergic conditions, supporting the immune and nervous system.

Marigold (*Calendula officinalis*):   Grows very easily from seed. Plant in small compost-filled pots and keep moist. Transplant outside at the end of Spring, after the last frost. Can also be sown from May onwards directly where you want them to flower. A sun-loving plant

- *Parts used:* flowers.
- *Good for:* reducing inflammation, wound healing, and antibacterial, antifungal, and antiviral activity, with strong antiseptic properties.

Milk thistle (*Silybum marianum/Carduus marianus*):   Grows well, like a dandelion, from seed; plant after last frost; can grow to a height of 3 m; wear gloves to harvest seeds in the summer.

- *Parts used:* seeds.
- *Good for:* protecting the liver from toxins, drugs, alcohol, and viruses; supporting detoxification process in the body.

Sweet wormwood (*Artemisia annua*):   Grows well from seed and is a very fast-growing plant. Sweet wormwood is best planted at the back of the garden, as it can reach a height of 1.8 m. It prefers a sunny position in well-drained soil.

- *Parts used:* leaves and stalks.
- *Good for:* its antiparasitic and antifungal activity.

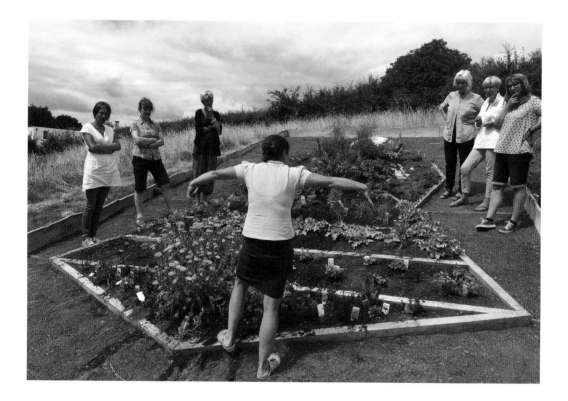

Valerian (*Valeriana officinalis*):   Extremely hardy; in full bloom it is a strongly scented plant that grows up to 1.8 m tall. You can grow valerian from seed or buy a plant from a nursery.

- *Parts used:* roots.
- *Good for:* reducing anxiety, stress-related conditions such as insomnia, neck pain, headaches, muscle cramps, irritability, stomach ache, irritable bowel syndrome.

There are many other herbs that are easy to grow and beneficial to wellbeing, including calendula, dandelion, lavender, thyme, St John's wort, lemon balm, sage, and garlic.

Harvesting

Harvesting is a simple process, but there are a few considerations to ensure the maximum quality of the herb and to preserve the health of the plants. Using a sharp knife or a pair of garden scissors, harvest small amounts of herb, to use fresh in infusions and enliven your cooking. Rosemary and mint, in particular, add a wonderful aromatic overtone to dishes. Harvest herbs to dry, preferably on a sunny day, in general between mid-morning and noon. Never harvest more than one-third of a plant at a time, and allow young plants to re-grow before harvesting from them again.

Drying leaves

You can tie 6–8 stems together and hang in an airy, dry place. Leave until completely dry, before pulling off the leaves and storing in a paper bag or glass jar, in a cool, dark place.

You can also dry in a dehydrator. Cut the leaves from the stem and lay them on a dehydrator drying tray, trying not to overlap. Dry as close to a temperature of 30°C as possible, until the leaves are dry and crumble easily between the fingers, then cool, and store.

Drying flowers

Spread flowers evenly on clean paper and leave to dry in a not-too-warm, airy place, away from direct sunlight; this should take 4 to 5 days. Store in paper bags or glass jars in a cool, dark place. Alternatively, use a dehydrator, as described above.

Drying plant roots

Most roots should be harvested in the plant's second year; as they get older than that, they become more fibrous and woody. In general, roots for drying are dug in the autumn. Harvest the roots, gently easing them

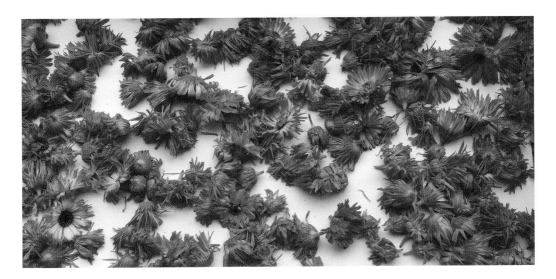

from the soil with a fork. Rinse them under cool running water, using a soft brush to clean off all the dirt. Chop into small pieces and dry in a dehydrator or oven at 50°C, until hard and crisp. Cool before packing in an airtight container, and store in a cool, dark place.

Be sure to label containers clearly.

You can also preserve herbs in honey, vinegar, or alcohol, for use when they are no longer in season.

Trees to grow for the future

Trees provide us with a wonderful opportunity to connect with nature: they attract insects and garden birds, as well as giving a glorious display of foliage and blossom. Trees are the "lungs of the planet". We rely on their photosynthesising power to absorb greenhouse gases and to help to counter climate change. Trees also provide us with food and powerful medicine. Being with/under trees is an essential part of your recovery from Lyme disease. Every tree you plant will, in time, support your health and wellbeing as well as that of the planet and future generations.

Not everyone has a garden large enough to plant a tree – though some trees fare well in a container, or you could plant a tree in a community garden. Here are six trees for you to choose from: they are all very simple to source and plant, as well as being very low-maintenance. Any one of these trees will bring you great pleasure as you watch it grow and will support health in a myriad ways.

Ginkgo (*Ginkgo biloba*)

The ginkgo tree, which is native to China, dates back 200 million years, well before the dinosaurs. It is very adaptable and can grow in any temperate climate, eventually reaching a height of up to 30 m high and 9 m wide – so probably too big for most gardens! It would, however, be perfect to plant in a community space. It prefers dry or moist soil, can tolerate drought, but does not like growing in shade.

Ginkgo has a long history of medicinal use, especially in China. The cooked seeds are astringent and sedative and used in the treatment of asthma and coughs. Ginkgo leaves, which are harvested just as they

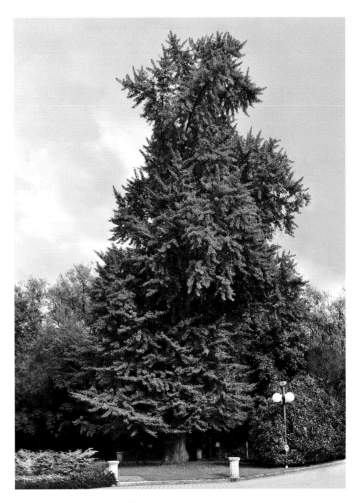

begin to turn yellow, have a range of medicinally active compounds that can reduce inflammation, increase circulation, and help to improve memory, concentration, and thought processes. Some studies have shown it to be beneficial in reducing depression, PMS symptoms, and sexual dysfunction.[1]

Hawthorn (*Crataegus monogyna*)

Hawthorn is often called "Tree of the Heart". This fast-growing tree is found throughout Britain, Europe, and parts of North America.

A single tree can grow to 10 m, but hawthorn has long been grown as a hedging plant. The delicate green leaves, often the first to appear in

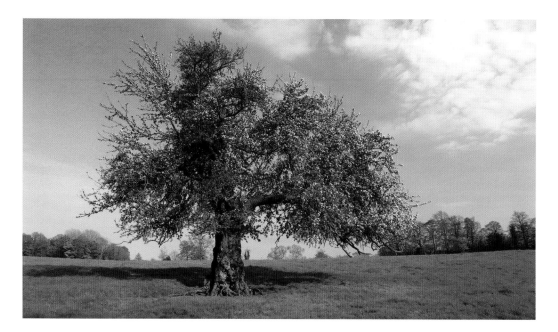

spring, are followed by a dazzling display of pretty blossom. The dense branches make a perfect nesting shelter for many birds.

The young leaves, flower buds, and young flowers are all edible and can be added to green salads. The berries, known as haws, are commonly used to make jellies and wines.

The haws, leaves, and flowers, in tinctures, powder, or teas, are used to strengthen and improve heart function and to help to reduce blood pressure.

Olive (*Olea europaea*)

The olive tree is central to the culture of Mediterranean countries. It is extremely long lived, but it does not grow particularly large – no taller than 15 m. It needs hot weather, is drought tolerant, and can withstand a light frost. In cold or northern regions, olive trees can be grown in containers that can be brought inside for protection in the winter. Olive trees grown in a container will need regular watering and feeding to produce fruit. Olives and their oil are rich in vitamin E, iron, copper, and beneficial monounsaturated fat.

Olive tree leaves have antioxidant and anti-inflammatory benefits and can be used in a tea or as an extract or powder.

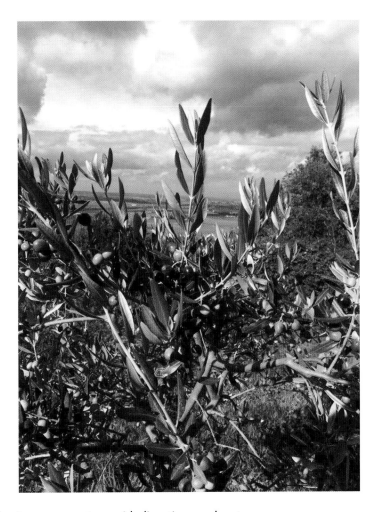

The leaves can boost the immune system, aid digestion, and act as a cardiac tonic; they have antifungal, antiviral, anti-mycoplasma, and pain-relieving properties. The olive tree is evergreen, and a simple, calming tea can be made all year round from the leaves.

Silver birch (*Betula alba*)

Silver birches are fast-growing, slender, upright trees with a silvery white bark. The tree grows throughout Northern Europe. It is very hardy and tolerates cold conditions. It is a popular garden tree and very easy to grow. Woodpeckers often nest in the trunk, and greenfinches visit to eat the seeds. In early Celtic mythology the birch symbolised purification and

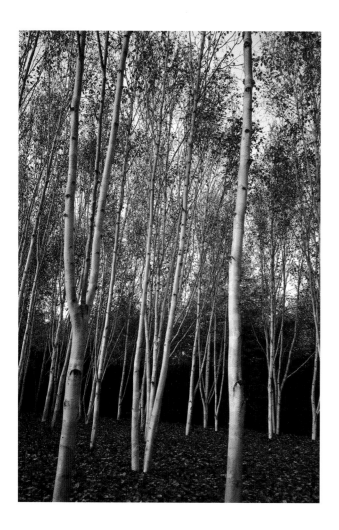

renewal. Twigs were used to remove negative energies. The sap can be collected from mature trees and used as a sugar substitute; it also has an antiseptic effect on the urinary system.

Birch leaves are antiseptic and used as an infusion. The young leaves are a gentle sedative. The healing properties of birch bark and birch bark extracts have been known for a long time. The phytochemicals in the bark have anti-inflammatory, antimicrobial, antiviral, and antioxidant activity and can be beneficial in supporting the immune system. Recent studies have found that betulin, a compound in silver birch bark, can help to prevent Type 2 diabetes.

White willow (*Salix alba*)

White willow is the largest of the willow trees; it can be found growing throughout the northern hemisphere. It can grow up to 25 m tall, so it needs a large garden. White willow likes wet ground and is often found growing near rivers and streams. The catkins are an early source of nectar and pollen for bees.

White willow bark has long been used as a powerful pain relief remedy.

Willow's active chemical constituent – salicin – was identified in 1829. It is a powerful anti-inflammatory and analgesic that relieves inflammation and pain without the side effects often caused by over-the-counter medication like ibuprofen. Willow bark promotes blood flow and reduces swelling, soothing menstrual cramps, muscle pain, and arthritis.

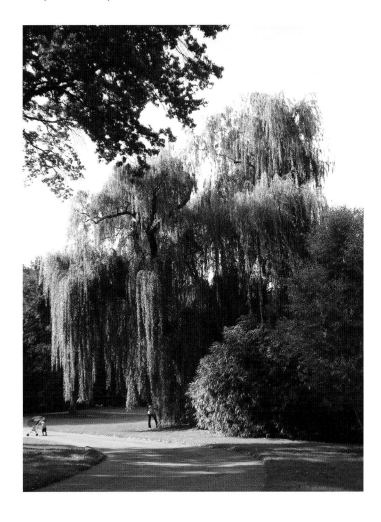

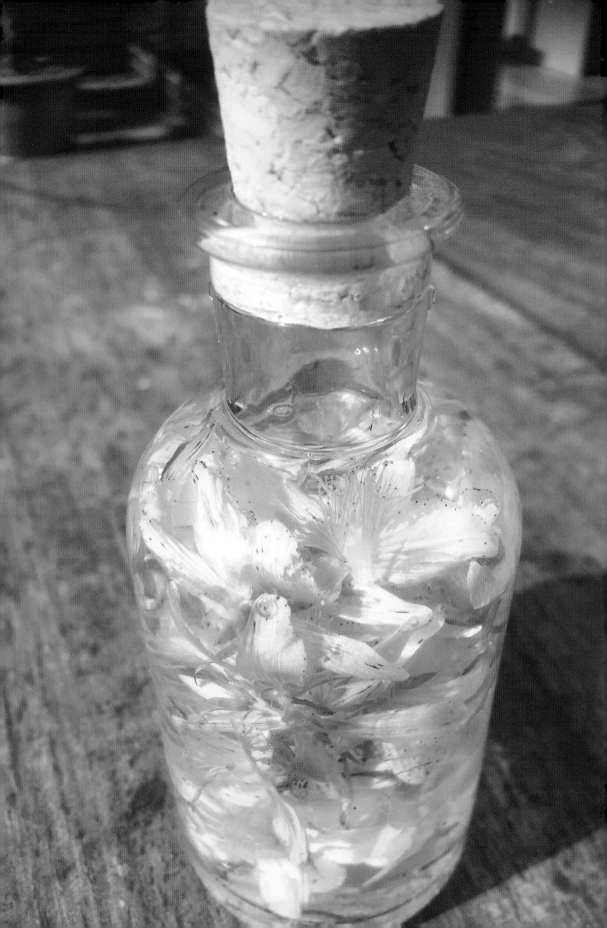

10

For practitioners

Figures suggest that there is an increasing number of cases of Lyme disease in the United Kingdom. But the figures could be too low and actually be three times higher than estimated, *at around 8,000,* in 2019. In the United States 300,000 new cases were estimated between 2005 and 2010.[1] These numbers were updated in 2015, with a revised figure of a 320% increase.[2]

The growing incidence of Lyme disease is due in part to changes in the weather and also to the increase in travel and change in habits of the vector – the tick. Not just deer, but also rodents, family pets, and birds are able to carry ticks. Birds can spread tick-borne illness wherever they fly. So there is a great likelihood that you will find that more and more people come to you with Lyme disease.

Herbal practitioners provide an environment of care within which the client is able to develop self-care and find the tools they need to heal. A herbal medical practitioner with a patient-centred approach will need to revisit everything they have ever learned. Clinical training and examination techniques will be invaluable. All practitioners should be aware of the debilitating signs and complexities in the symptoms of Lyme disease. You will need to expand your knowledge in differential diagnosis with unfamiliar multifactorial ailments, identification, and red flags.

It is also important to build up a team of experts to refer to. If you do not want to draw blood or become a phlebotomist, then find one. You will need blood tests and results to support you and your client in order to find your clinical approach. Different practitioners and methods will vary, depending on the country in which you live or work.

Often people think Lyme disease is just one infection treated by antibiotics; they are often surprised to hear about co-infections and the overlapping of clinical manifestations resembling other illnesses arising from bacteria, viruses, and mould. The more tests you do, the more clinical findings become apparent. The virus often complicates healing, as do unresolved sexually transmitted illnesses that had not been picked up before.

Having had Lyme disease and having recovered from the infection does not give lifelong immunity: it is possible to be reinfected and develop Lyme disease again.

There are many overlapping symptoms that can be helped with herbs. But there is not one magic formula or pill that will fix all. Many of your clients want answers when there are just more questions, and clear directions when there are many options. Supporting people with Lyme disease is complex and time-consuming – a commitment to your client, research, and the process of healing.

It can take anywhere from 7 days to 2 years to see improvement with your patient, and longer when Lyme disease is chronic. If you are unable to commit to this, make sure you are able to give a referral to someone who can offer long-term support.

Often patients' past experiences have been traumatic, and they need support in order to help build strength for healing. I normally allow two hours for a consultation, so the client feels they have had an opportunity to share their story and there is time for an exchange of information.

The key I have found to helping my clients is listening, encouraging people to share their stories, unlocking the door that holds the pain, their experience so far, and then identifying the tools they will need to move on. Finding out what is important to your client is important for them to reach their goals of wellbeing.

Before you meet your first Lyme patient, make sure you are well versed in the subject and have had at least 10 years' clinical experience as a herbal practitioner. Also be prepared for your client to know a lot more about their condition than you do at first.

First meeting

When, as a therapist, you see the patient for the first time, you may need to explain what you do, and the setup of your practice: whether you are an individual in private practice supporting people with Lyme disease or are part of an integrated health practice. Tell them that you will take a detailed case history, and that you may have to organise some blood tests and do an examination to determine how to proceed with treatment. You may also explain how long this may take. This is an important part of documenting patient care and will help the patient to understand how you will both work together to create a care plan unique to the individual.

Take down a detailed case history, including:

- demographic information
- chief complaint, and current level of activity
- patient goals
- prior level of functioning
- social history and cultural beliefs
- employment history
- family and medical history
- other health care professionals they rely on and other diagnostic information

If they do require further tests, be prepared, as you may need to direct them to people you work with who can do this. Having a list of labs that your client can be referred to will be beneficial to the client. You may, however, need to explain that not all blood tests are 100% reliable in the diagnosis of Lyme disease.

After an initial conversation, schedule a Zoom call or face-to-face consultation, allowing plenty of time. Ensure that they have filled in and returned to you, prior to consultation, all the following:

- brief record of past medical history
- results of any recent or relevant tests
- medical history and relevant surgery that has affected their health
- a three-day food diary
- a list of any medication and supplements they are taking
- a list of any antibiotics they have used, and for how long

Diagnosis

Establish the potential symptoms of Lyme disease. Richard Horowitz, a New York Lyme specialist, uses a questionnaire that was developed by Joseph Burrascano to determine the likelihood of Lyme disease. Getting patients to fill in this questionnaire can help to indicate how likely it is that they are suffering from a tick-borne infection.[3] (Also see description of bull's-eye rash in chapters 1 and 3.)

Note that because Lyme disease can inhibit the immune system, patients can also have a false-negative antibody test. According to a recent paper,[4] 11 people with a negative ELISA at a London hospital were nevertheless sent for a Western blot, and of the 11, 6 had a positive Western blot.

SYMPTOMS OF LYME DISEASE

Please highlight or tick all symptoms you are experiencing but be aware they may not be symptoms of Lyme disease.

☐ Unexplained fevers, sweats, chills or flushing

☐ Unexplained weight change: loss or gain

☐ Fatigue, tiredness

☐ Unexplained hair loss

☐ Swollen glands

☐ Sore throat

☐ Testicular pain or pelvic pain

☐ Unexplained menstrual irregularity

☐ Unexplained milk production and/or breast pain

☐ Irritable bladder or bladder dysfunction

☐ Sexual dysfunction or loss of libido

☐ Upset stomach

☐ Change in bowel function: constipation or diarrhea

☐ Chest pain or rib soreness

☐ Shortness of breath, cough

☐ Heart palpitations, pulse skips, heart block

☐ History of a heart murmur or valve prolapse

☐ Joint pain or swelling – please list joints:

☐ Stiffness of the joints, neck or back

☐ Muscle pain or cramps

☐ Twitching of the face or other muscles

☐ Headaches

☐ Neck aches; neck stiffness

☐ Tingling, numbness, burning or stabbing sensations

☐ Facial paralysis (Bells Palsy)

☐ Eyes/vision: double, blurry

☐ Ears/hearing: buzzing, ringing, ear pain

☐ Increased motion sickness, vertigo

☐ Lightheadedness, wooziness, poor balance, difficulty walking

☐ Tremors

☐ Confusion, difficulty thinking

☐ Difficulty with concentration or reading

☐ Forgetfulness, poor short term memory

☐ Disorientation: getting lost, going to the wrong places

☐ Difficulty with speech or writing

☐ Mood swings, irritability, depression

☐ Disturbed sleep – too much or too little or early awakening

☐ Exaggerated symptoms or worse hangover from alcohol

Lyme disease symptoms questionnaire.

Treatment

In my experience, Lyme clients are the most absorbing of all clients; maintaining friendly boundaries is important for all concerned. Even though you want to give support in any way you can, you can also be overtaken by the needs of the client.

Really listen, so you are able to understand where someone is coming from. Just as important as the herbs that you give is being a compassionate listener. You might be the only person they have shared some of their life experiences with.

Clients often take a range of herbs. As my clients are already taking a huge variety of supplements when they see me, I might use a 5:1 concentrated preparation of Japanese knotweed or Chinese skullcap; I leave for later the tincture for heat-decocted cat's claw (*U. tomentosa*) and other herbs specific for that individual's needs.

Many clients want a breakdown of herbs and information sent with herbs, or followed up with an e-mail. The follow-up notes are particularly helpful for the client to see their progress: as people can remember events differently, notes help you remind your clients how things have improved. These notes should include:

  ▷ a follow-up form (to be filled out before each visit)
  ▷ ArminLabs checklist form
  ▷ a list of phlebotomists to draw blood, if needed
  ▷ the price list

One can follow broad guidelines and protocols that have been developed over many years by various clinics and Lyme specialists, but health outcomes can be improved by using herbal medicine and making nutritional changes.

Do not underestimate the many other emotional, physical, and social factors that can influence the eventual outcome of overall health. Factor in that treatments can go on for years and need to be adapted as the condition and client changes.

Notes around dosing

  ▷ Doses will depend on individual effective detox pathways: some of my clients with small frames can actually cope with much higher doses, while others start with drop dose.

> ▷ I often start with a low dose and build up slowly. I have various pre-prepared dropper bottles to speed dispensing, as larger or complex prescriptions may take some time to prepare.
> ▷ Gut health is a huge factor in the speed of increasing the dosage: for example, in my experience, clients can struggle with taking mushrooms if they have a sensitive digestive tract, particularly if there is a history of antibiotic use.

Most Lyme clients go on to lead a normal life, but others may lack the motivation. Sometimes I buddy up clients or parents so they can give each other the support and success stories they need to keep each other motivated. Daphne Lambert's retreats enable people to share their stories. Sometimes there is a fear of being unique and different. I am struck by the under-acknowledgement the effect of Lyme disease is having on people: the sharing of journeys enables the successes to come to the surface.

And do remember: as a practitioner, it is important to be aware of your own health and the demands placed on you by your clients. You are just as much at risk of burn-out and physical exhaustion if you are not making time for yourself.

An Australian client of mine had been through hell. She came to England in search of help. She had been given electric shock treatment for depression again and again before she came here and got the combination of antibiotics and herbal medicine treatment she needed.[5] She went from not being able to read more than a few lines due to Borrelia bacteria causing blurred vision, fatigue, and brain fog to eventually being able to read freely and write her own book.

> "I got quite a bit better as a result of taking the Byron White herbs. But things plateaued – like a hill I could not quite get to the top of. Two things seemed to make a difference to me: antiparasitic treatment and dental hygiene. My gums and teeth did not fare well with Lyme disease. I eventually had a tooth removed, and things strongly improved.
>
> I am not spending much on treatment nowadays: small expenditure on managing cold sores and the herpes virus."

Working with children

One of the first clients who ever came to see me had recovered well from Lyme disease, but when she became pregnant a few years later, she was afraid she may still be carrying a dormant form and pass it on to her unborn baby. It is at times like this that you need doctors, experts, and colleagues who can reassure expectant mothers. This is not the sort of work you can do without a team.

Some parents with Lyme disease fear they might have passed it on to their children, or that their children have got Lyme disease from playing in the fields. Others feel their children have Lyme disease when they are not developing as the parents feel they should be.

Diagnosing Lyme disease is also, frankly, impossible when children are too young to talk, or they live overseas and you are asked to help on a screen, especially when there has been no bull's-eye rash or history of tick bite.

When you are taking on a client with Lyme disease, you have to consider the whole family. It is important to hear directly from the child how they are feeling, rather than purely letting the parent speak. Often you may find yourself, as a practitioner, the bridge of deeper healing, facilitating, and creating new links in family chains.

A teenager, whose mother was a cardiac surgeon, was referred to see me. I prescribed herbs, and within a year his symptoms had improved and his retesting came back negative. I noticed that even though he was pleased with the outcome, he still craved the love of his parent, and it was this that seemed to inhibit his full recovery. Over the year, while exploring healing opportunities, it became apparent that the pain was much deeper and connected to the arrival of a new family member and changing family dynamics. Each one-to-one session became an opportunity to discuss the pain within the family dynamics. This did not improve until a meeting was held with both parent and child, giving an opportunity for feelings to be heard. I could not help wonder how the child's sickness had helped him gain the care he needed from a parent who was normally quite distracted by their own work.

It can be hard responding to your child's feelings if you see things differently in their behaviour and actions. For example, a girl who came to see me with her mother said she had awful headaches, brain fog, dizziness, and nauseous pain all over; in the last few days she had thought she was going to die. She was taken to hospital. They did numerous tests, but everything came back negative. She was desperate to find out what was going on in her body.

From the mother's perspective, her daughter's health was improving, and she was going out more. Only the day before, she had done 50 sit-ups, taken the dog for a walk, and played the piano for two hours. But the daughter had immersed herself in the thought that things had not improved, rather than acknowledging the things that had.

Her feelings were real; denying them might have led to alienation and slow recovery. We all know how we can feel so much better when our feelings are validated and understood. A child has not had all the experiences we have had, and lessons in resilience that go with the aging process.

Some people are ultra-sensitive to their environment, and this can have a huge impact on their health; others may naturally be more robust and keen to take on new ideas.

Children, like adults, respond to their environment and the people they meet.

As children, we learn to manage our feelings, often guided by our parents. Those feelings may be taken seriously by the parent in order to keep the child safe, or they may be dismissed. When a child's needs are not being met or heard, this can lead to behavioural issues of anxiety or depression. Whether this is the illness part of a Lyme picture or a different diagnosis, it is important to get the right help.

If you are working with children under 16, you are likely to be working with a paediatrician or a therapist who specialises in working with children.

Developmental changes, symptoms, and blood results might be quite different from those of adults. According to some paediatric doctors that I spoke to in Germany at a Lyme conference, CD57 might be low in children and not indicate an infection, as their immune systems are just developing.

For some children there may be similarities between autism spectrum disorders, neurological disorders, and Lyme disease. Speech and learning can be affected with children with Lyme disease, making it difficult to diagnose. When children with both Lyme disease and autism are given Lyme treatment, their autism may improve.

Practitioners in the Lyme-light

This is an evolving field: no single expert has all the answers, so we must look at a broad spectrum of approaches to find solutions. The following are some the most prominent practitioners in the field of Lyme disease.

Stephen Harrod Buhner [1952–2022]: American herbalist and cutting-edge researcher in herbal medicine and the author of over 23 award-winning books: *Healing Lyme: Natural Healing of Lyme Borreliosis and the Coinfections Chlamydia and Spotted Fever Rickettsiosis, Healing Lyme Disease Coinfections: Complementary and Holistic Treatments for Bartonella and Mycoplasma,* and *Herbal Antivirals: Natural Remedies For Emerging & Resistant Viral Infections,* all aimed at health care professionals and their patients.

Without his extensive work and experience as a practitioner, I would not have known were to begin. His books have guided my understanding of Lyme and are very user-friendly. He had a holistic-centred approach and was well versed in herbs, supplements, and mushrooms. His work is essential reading.

Lee Cowden, MD: Practised integrative medicine for 30 years before retiring to pursue full-time teaching. In his experience, people with chronic illness may have Lyme disease. He has created a complex 9-month protocol using drop doses of 14 different supplements. He also recommends avoiding electromagnetic radiation, eating a raw, organic diet, and reducing allergens and processed foods. (https://drleecowden.com/project/csp-lyme)

Richard Horowitz, MD: American medical doctor and director of the Hudson Valley Healing Arts Center. He has supported thousands of people with Lyme disease with a combination of orthodox medicine and complementary treatments. He is an advocate of the Byron White Formulas, which are designed to support Lyme and co-infections. (Byron White Formulas are used by many health care practitioners to detox, restore, and support the immune system. I sometimes use these when symptoms plateau, and I have had a number of clients who find them very useful.)

His book, *Why Can't I Get Better? Solving the Mystery of Lyme and Chronic Disease,* was published in 2013. He uses the MSIDS [Multiple Systemic Infectious Disease] model to describe Lyme disease and how co-infections can cause persistent illness in patients, causing immune dysfunction and inflammation, and showing that there are many great imitators of Lyme disease and that regulating sugar levels, detoxifying with glutathione, and the effect of mould should not be overlooked when supporting people with Lyme disease.

Dietrich Klinghardt: German medical doctor specialising in chronic conditions, working in the United Kingdom, Europe, and the United States. He talks of different levels of healing: treating what we see under a microscope, and the personal trauma that has affected our genetic makeup. He has also done some interesting work related to mould, chemical sensitivity, and electromagnetic stressors in our environment from everyday products that could be responsible for chronic illness. (https://klinghardtinstitute.com)

Epilogue

Healing Lyme disease is not a linear journey: it goes in multiple directions. In reading this book, I trust you have found a far greater understanding of the complications and complexities of Lyme, the overlapping nature of co-infections, and how our responses have a massive impact on healing.

The language we use to describe health, couched, as it is, in war termi-nology, is not helpful: combatting illness, surviving Lyme disease, fighting a battle. It puts us into victim mode rather than empowering us to take health into our own hands.

I often hear people say, "if only I did this" and "if only I did that". But with this approach we can spiral into a negative loop, when actually we need to be looking for options and ways to support ourselves, finding tools and answers rather than looking for stumbling blocks. Working with medicinal plants for over 20 years has shown me that nature holds many of the answers we are looking for.

The stories I hear are all different, but they share a common thread of being lost in an unfamiliar land, struggling to find a way home. My wish for those with Lyme is that this book helps you to find the path. *Lost in Lyme* is an invitation to think positively in respect of Lyme, with an image in your mind of a friend, to believe in your power to restore wellbeing, to learn to use nature's medicinal plants, and to be kind to yourself as you travel the road ahead, picking knowledge from the plants on your way.

Final quote to encourage you to be confident in your recovery

"For me, after years of illness the initial treatment following diagnosis was fantastic, I saw a 70% improvement in about 3 months. After that, things plateaued, but I kept on with the treatment, always wanting 100%. Eventually the Dr (that Julia works with) told me to stop – I wanted to continue, desperate for full recovery. After a treatment break, I was given the Byron White regime – for me, it delivered a further step up in improvement, but still short of 100%. Again I hung on to the treatment, not wanting to stop, even though for many months it appeared to make no difference. Eventually I stopped all treatment – it felt like losing my security blanket. That was 7 years ago. The situation then was that I no longer felt ill (I used to feel as if I had been poisoned, really sick and unwell), but I still had some of the physical symptoms (tremors, muscle weakness, bad reaction to physical activity etc.).

Now for the good news ... recovery continued after treatment stopped, but so slowly over the years that I did not notice for a long time. Today I can do very much more than I could at the point treatment stopped. Even so, I still get the return of some physical symptoms; however, the time between the symptoms gets longer and longer, maybe 2 months with nothing, the symptoms are milder and last for less time, sometimes hours rather than days and, previously, weeks.

What is also important is that when the symptoms do recur, I now assume they will go away again; previously I panicked that it was all coming back. Lymes is a long, slow road, but you can recover. You may have to accept that some things cannot be fixed and will not return to pre-Lyme state, but also, as the years pass, age may come to play a part as well! Some symptoms will recur, but most likely it is your brain/nervous system delivering signals to your body that have been learned during Lyme with no 'underlying active Lyme cause'. That was the thought of the doctor who worked with Julia. Also, some things are not related to Lyme. For me, if I get any illness at all, my first thought is still that it is Lyme-related! A personal choice I made, which was helpful for me, was not to "Google" anything on Lyme – on the few occasions I did, the result was anxiety rather than knowledge/solutions, so I put my trust in Julia and the doctor."

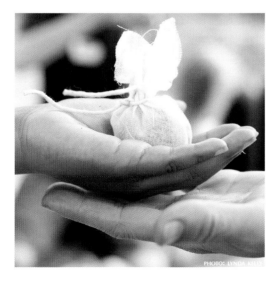
PHOTO: LYNDA KELLY

NOTES

Chapter 1

1. M. Davidsson, "The financial implications of a well-hidden and ignored chronic Lyme disease pandemic". *Healthcare (Basel), 6* (1) (2018): 16.
2. R. A. Sykes & P. Makiello, "An estimate of Lyme borreliosis incidence in Western Europe". *J. Public Health, 39* (2017): 74–81.
3. A Rizzoli, "Lyme borreliosis in Europe". *Eurosurveillance, 16* (27) (2011). https://www.eurosurveillance.org/content/10.2807/ese.16.27.19906-en; Z. Ji et al., "Prevalence of *Borrelia burgdorferi* in Ixodidae tick around Asia: A systematic review and meta-analysis". *Pathogens, 11* (2) (2022): 143; K. Kurtenbach et al., "Fundamental processes in the evolutionary ecology of Lyme borreliosis". *Nat. Rev. Microbiol., 4* (2006): 660–669.
4. CDC. *Lyme Disease Data Tables 2019: Historical Data.* https://www.cdc.gov/lyme/stats/humancases.html
5. X. Zhang et al., "Economic impact of Lyme disease". *Emerg. Infect. Dis., 12* (4) (2006): 653–660.
6. M. Wec & M. Lvh, "The bacteria of periodontal diseases". *Periodontol. 2000, 5* (1994): 66–77.

Chapter 2

1. https://www.nhs.uk/conditions/lyme-disease
2. M. Citera et al., "Empirical validation of the Horowitz Multiple Systemic Infectious Disease Syndrome Questionnaire for suspected Lyme disease". *Int. J. Gen. Med., 10* (2017): 249–273.
3. https://pathologytestsexplained.org.au/learning/test-index/antibody-tests
4. https://www.hindawi.com/journals/isrn/2012/719821
5. M. J. Cook & B. P. Puri, "Commercial test kits for detection of Lyme borreliosis: A meta-analysis of test accuracy". *Int. J. Gen. Med., 9* (2016): 427–440.
6. Ibid.
7. R. B. Stricker & L. Johnson, "Lyme disease: The promise of Big Data, companion diagnostics and precision medicine". *Infect. Drug Resist., 9* (2016): 215–219.
8. https://www.rosaliegreenbergmd.com/post/problems-with-present-lyme-disease-testing-how-individuals-especially-children-are-shortchanged
9. L. Meriläinen et al., "Morphological and biochemical features of *Borrelia burgdorferi* pleomorphic forms". *Microbiology (Reading), 161* (Pt 3) (2015): 516–527.
10. M. Sedegah, "The Ex Vivo IFN-γ Enzyme-Linked Immunospot (ELISpot) Assay". In: A. Vaughan (Ed.), *Malaria Vaccines: Methods and Protocols* (New York: Humana Press, 2018), 3rd edition, pp. 197–205.

11. https://aonm.org/armin-labs/tests/elispot
12. J. Dunaj et al., "The role of PCR in diagnostics of Lyme borreliosis". *Przegl. Epidemiol., 67* (1) (2013): 35–39, 119–23.
13. https://www.immunology.org/public-information/bitesized-immunology/receptors-molecules/immunoglobulin-iga
14. R. Dillon et al., "Lyme disease in the U.K.: Clinical and laboratory features and response to treatment". *Clin. Med. (Lond.), 10* (5) (2010): 454–457.

Chapter 3

1. https://www.cdc.gov/lyme/prev/vaccine.html
2. S. H. Buhner, *Healing Lyme: Natural Healing of Lyme Borreliosis and the Coinfections Chlamydia and Spotted Fever Rickettsiosis, 2nd edition* (Randolph, VT: Raven Press, 2015), p. 211.
3. R. Horowitz, *Why Can't I Get Better? Solving the Mystery of Lyme and Chronic Disease* (New York: St Martin's Press, 2013).
4. https://lymeconnection.org/support_and_resources/meet_the_lyme_disease_experts.html/title/dr-richard-horowitz-latest-treatments-in-lyme-disease
5. M. Laszkowska et al., "Nationwide population-based cohort study of celiac disease and risk of Ehlers–Danlos syndrome and joint hypermobility syndrome. *Dig. Liver Dis., 48* (9) (2016): 1030–1034.
6. https://klinghardtinstitute.com/wp-content/uploads/2020/06/Lyme-Co-infections-Protocol-May-2020.pdf

Chapter 4

1 M. T. Melia & P. G. Auwaerter, "Time for a different approach to Lyme disease and long-term symptoms". *N. Engl. J. Med., 374* (2016): 1277–1278.
2. https://www.lymedisease.org/horowitz-dapsone-chronic-lyme/
3. C.-Y. Huang et al., "Hyperbaric oxygen therapy as an effective adjunctive treatment for chronic Lyme disease". *J. Chinese Med. Assoc., 77* (5) (2014): 269–271,
4. S. K. Pavelić et al., "Critical review on Zeolite Clinoptilolite safety and medical applications *in vivo*". *Front. Pharmacol, 9* (2018): 1350.
5. R. Ben-Ami et al., "Antibiotic exposure as a risk factor for fluconazole-resistant Candida Bloodstream infection". *Antimicrob. Agents Chemother., 56* (5) (2012): 2518–2523.
6. B. S. Park et al., "Curcuma longa L. constituents inhibit sortase A and Staphylococcus aureus cell adhesion to fibronectin". *J. Agric. Food Chem., 53* (23) (2005): 9005–9009.
8. C. Etheridge (2016), *Mechanisms of Antibacterial Herbal Action* (http://ehtpa.org/pdf/Mechanisms%20of%20antibacterial%20herbal%20action%20-%20handout.pdf); K. Karaosmanoglu et al.. "Assessment of berberine as a multi-target antimicrobial: A multi-omics study for drug discovery and repositioning". *OMICS., 18*(1) (2014): 42–53; A. V. Anand et al., "Medicinal plants, phytochemicals, and herbs to combat viral pathogens including SARS-CoV-2". *Molecules, 26* (6) (2021): 1775.
9. Wittschier et al., "Aqueous extracts and polysaccharides from liquorice roots (Glycyrrhiza glabra L.) inhibit adhesion of Helicobacter pylori to human gastric mucosa". *J. Ethnopharmacol., 125* (2) (2009): 218–223.
10. A. Ramirez-Hernandez et al., "Adherence reduction of *Campylobacter jejuni* and

Campylobacter coli strains to HEp-2 Cells by Mannan oligosaccharides and a high-molecular-weight component of cranberry extract". *J. Food Protect., 78* (8) (2015): 1496–1505; K. L. Kaspar et al., "A randomized, double-blind, placebo-controlled trial to assess the bacterial anti-adhesion effects of cranberry extract beverages". *FoodFunct., 6* (2015): 1212–1217.

11. H.-H. Yu et al., "Antimicrobial activity of berberine alone and in combination with ampicillin or oxacillin against methicillin-resistant Staphylococcus aureus". *J. Med. Food., 8* (4) (2005): 454–461.

12. S. H. Buhner, *Healing Lyme Disease Coinfections: Complementary and Holistic Treatments for Bartonella and Mycoplasma* (Rochester, VT: Healing Arts Press, 2013).

13. A. Klančnik et al., "Rosemary resistant Campylobacter jejuni, restoring susceptibility to various antibiotics". *PLoS One, 7* (12) (2012): e51800.

14. M. Stavri et al., "Bacterial efflux pump inhibitors from natural sources". *J. Antimicrob. Chemother., 59* (6) (2007): 1247–1260.

15. Khameneh, B. et al., "Review on plant antimicrobials: A mechanistic viewpoint". *Antimicrob. Resist. Infect. Control, 8* (2019): 118.

16. R. Quinn, "Rethinking antibiotic research and development: World War II and the penicillin collaborative". *Am. J. Public Health, 103* (3) (2012): 426–434.

17. H. Kawagishi & C. Zhuang, "Compounds for dementia from Hericium erinaceum". *Drugs Future, 33* (2008): 149–155.

18. S. H. Buhner, *Healing Lyme: Natural Healing of Lyme Borreliosis and the Coinfections Chlamydia and Spotted Fever Rickettsiosis, 2nd Edition* (Randolph, VT: Raven Press, 2015), pp. 276–278.

19. J. Feng et al., "Evaluation of natural and botanical medicines for activity against growing and non-growing forms of B. burgdorferi". *Front. Med. (Lausanne), 7* (2020): 6.

20. Buhner, *Healing Lyme.*

Chapter 5

1. S. Kasture et al., "Withania somnifera prevents morphine withdrawal-induced decrease in spine density in nucleus accumbens shell of rats: A confocal laser scanning microscopy study". *Neurotox. Res., 16* (4) (2009): 343–355.

2. K. Bone & S. Mills (Eds.), *Principles and Practice of Phytotherapy: Modern Herbal Medicine, 2nd Edition* (New York: Elsevier, 2012).

3. S. H. Buhner, *Healing Lyme: Natural Healing of Lyme Borreliosis and the Coinfections Chlamydia and Spotted Fever Rickettsiosis, 2nd Edition* (Randolph, VT: Raven Press, 2015), p. 278.

4. Ibid., p. 388.

5. Ibid.

6. Y. J. Hsu et al., "Anti-hyperglycemic effects and mechanism of Bidens pilosa water extract". *J. Ethnopharmacol., 122* (2) (2009): 379–383; T. Y. Jang et al., "Anti-allergic effect of luteolin in mice with allergic asthma and rhinitis". *Central European J. Immunol., 42* (1) (2017): 24–29; M. E. M. Camargo et al., "Diuretic effect of the aqueous extract of *Bidens odorata* in the rat". *J. Ethnopharmacol., 95* (2–3) (2004): 363–366; P. Sundararajan et al., "Studies of anticancer and antipyretic activity of *Bidens pilosa* whole plant". *Afr. Health Sci., 6* (1) (2006): 27–30.

7. X. Feng et al., "Berberine in cardiovascular and metabolic diseases: From mechanisms to therapeutics". *Theranostics., 9* (7) (2019): 1923–1951.

8. L. Lauk et al., "Activity of *Berberis aetensis* root extract on *candida* strains". *Fitoterapia, 78* (2) (2007): 159–161.
9. L. Slobodnikova et al., "Antimicrobial activity of Mahonia aquifolium crude extract and its major isolated alkaloids". *Phytother. Res., 18* (8) (2004): 674–676.
10. H.-H. Yu et al., "Antimicrobial activity of berberine alone and in combination with ampicillin or oxacillin against methicillin-resistant Staphylococcus aureus". *J. Med. Food., 8* (4) (2005): 454–461.
11. M. Cernáková & D. Kostálová, "Antimicrobial activity of berberine—a constituent of Mahonia aquifolium". *Folia. Microbiol. (Prague), 47* (4) (2002): 375–378.
12. H.-H. Yu et al., "Antimicrobial activity of berberine alone and in combination with ampicillin or oxacillin against methicillin-resistant Staphylococcus aureus". *J. Med. Food., 8* (4) (2005): 454–461.
13. S. H. Buhner, *Healing Lyme Disease Coinfections: Complementary and Holistic Treatments for Bartonella and Mycoplasma* (Rochester, VT: Healing Arts Press, 2013).
14. D. D. Li et al., "Fluconazole assists berberine to kill fluconazole-resistant *Candida albicans*". *Antimicrob. Agents Chemother., 57* (12) (2013): 6016–6027.
15. Y. X. Ni et al., "Therapeutic effect of berberine on 60 patients with non-insulin dependent diabetes mellitus and experimental research". *Chinese J. Integr. Tradition. Western Med., 1* (2) (1995): 91–95.
16. X. Zhang et al., "Structural changes of gut microbiota during berberine-mediated prevention of obesity and insulin resistance in high-fat diet-fed rats". *PLoS One, 7* (8) (2012): e42529.
17. Y. Hu et al., "Lipid-lowering effect of berberine in human subjects and rats". *Phytomed., 19* (10) (2012): 861–867.
18. Y. Li et al., "Letrozole, berberine, or their combination for anovulatory infertility in women with polycystic ovary syndrome: study design of a double-blind randomised controlled trial". *BMJ Open, 3* (2013): e003934.
19. Y. Ye et al., "Efficacy and safety of berberine alone for several metabolic disorders: A systematic review and meta-analysis of randomized clinical trials". *Front. Pharmacol., 12* (2021): 653887.
20. Lu et al. "Therapeutic effects of berberine on liver fibrosis are associated with lipid metabolism and intestinal flora". Front. Pharmacol., 13 (2022): 814871.
21. S. Mills & K. Bone, *The Essential Guide to Herbal Safety* (St Louis, MI: Elsevier, 2005).
22. S. Arthur, "The effectiveness of Samento, Cumanda, Burbur, and Dr. Lee Cowden's protocol in the treatment of chronic Lyme disease". *Townsend Letter: The Examiner of Alternative Medicine, 285* (2007).
23 J. Piscoya et al., "Efficacy and safety of freeze-dried cat's claw in osteoarthritis of the knee: Mechanisms of action of the species Uncaria guianensis". *Inflamm. Res., 50* (9) (2001): 442–448.
24. https://www.ncbi.nlm.nih.gov/pmc/articles/PMC5031759/#!po=0.694444
25. M.M. Iwu, *Handbook of African Medicinal Plants* (Boca Raton, FL: CRC Press, 2014).
26. I. Ben-Zvi et al., "Hydroxychloroquine: From malaria to autoimmunity". *Clin. Rev. Allergy Immunol., 42* (2) (2012): 145–153.
27. R. Hänsel & H. Haas, *Therapy with Phytopharmaceuticals* (Hailsham: School of Phytotherapy, 1997).
28. https://www.legislation.gov.uk/uksi/1977/2130/made
29. A. Hamilton, *Jesuit's Bark: A Reliable Medicine of Old with Surprising Current Controversy* (Lecture to West Sussex History of Medicine Society, MNIMH, 13 November 2021).
30. J. Feng et al., "Selective essential oils from spice or culinary herbs have high activity

against stationary phase and biofilm *Borrelia burgdorferi*". *Front. Med. (Lausanne), 4* (2017): 169.

31. "Ethnobotanical medicine is effective against the bacterium causing Lyme disease". *Featured News, Health,* 21 February 2020.

32. J. Feng et al., "Evaluation of natural and botanical medicines for activity against growing and non-growing forms of B. burgdorferi". *Front. Med. (Lausanne), 7* (2020): 6.

33. D. S. Oskouei et al., "The effect of Ginkgo biloba on functional outcome of patients with acute ischemic stroke: A double-blind, placebo-controlled, randomized clinical trial". *J. Stroke Cerebrovasc. Dis., 22* (8) (2013): e557–563.

34. A. von Boetticher, "Ginkgo biloba extract in the treatment of tinnitus: A systematic review". *Neuropsychiatr. Dis. Treat., 7* (2011): 441–447.

35. Buhner, *Healing Lyme,* p. 404.

36. Ibid., pp. 213–216, 336–353.

37. M. Z. El-Readi et al., "Fallopia japonica: Bioactive secondary metabolites and molecular mode of anticancer". *J. Trad. Med. Clin. Natur., 5* (2016): 193; C. K. Singh et al., "Resveratrol-based combinatorial strategies for cancer management". *Ann. NY Acad, Sci., 1290* (1) (2013): 113–121; M. H. Aziz et al., "Cancer chemoprevention by resveratrol: In vitro and in vivo studies and the underlying mechanisms" [Review]. *Int. J. Oncol., 23* (1) (2003): 17–28.

38. N. Vargas-Mendoza et al., ""Hepatoprotective effect of silymarin". *World J. Hepatol., 6* (3) (2014): 144–149.

39. http://www.telegraph.co.uk/news/health/3568094/The-best-hangover-remedies-tested.html

40. H. F. Huseini et al., "The efficacy of Silybum marianum (L.) Gaertn. (silymarin) in the treatment of type II diabetes: A randomized, double-blind, placebo-controlled, clinical trial". *Phytother. Res., 20* (12) (2006): 1036–1039.

41. https://www.acupuncturetoday.com/mpacms/at/article.php?id=32313

42. H. W. Leber & S. Knauff, "Influence of silymarin on drug metabolizing enzymes in rat and man". *Arzneim. Forsch., 26* (8) 1976: 1603–1605.

43. K Wojtyniak et al., "Leonurus cardiaca L. (motherwort): A review of its phytochemistry and pharmacology". *Phytother. Res., 27* (8) (2013): 1115–1120.

44. Y.-J. Wang et al., "Ursolic acid attenuates lipopolysaccharide-induced cognitive deficits in mouse brain through suppressing p38/NF-κB mediated inflammatory pathways". *Neurobiol. Learn. Mem., 96* (2) (2011): 156–165.

45. S. H. Buhner, *Healing Lyme: Natural Healing of Lyme Borreliosis and the Coinfections Chlamydia and Spotted Fever Rickettsiosis, 2nd Edition* (Randolph, VT: Raven Press, 2015), p. 381.

46. L. Parkinson & R. Keast, "Oleocanthal, a phenolic derived from virgin olive oil: A review of the beneficial effects on inflammatory disease". *Int. J. Mol. Sci., 15* (7) (2014): 12323–12334.

47. Buhner, *Healing Lyme Disease Coinfections,* p. 187.

48. Ibid., p. 191.

49. Ibid., pp. 198–202.

50. *Sardinian Cistus Incanus: A Simple Treatment of Mmany – If Not Most – Chronic Illnesses.* (https://klinghardtinstitute.com/articles/sardinian-cistus-incanus)

51. Z. Pu et al., "Assessment of the anti-virulence potential of extracts from four plants used in traditional Chinese Medicine against multidrug-resistant pathogens". *BMC Complement. Med. Ther., 20* (1) (2020): 318.

52. A. Scheinin et al., "Turku sugar studies XVIII. Incidence of dental caries in relation to 1-year consumption of xylitol chewing gum". *Acta Odontologica Scand., 33* (5) (1975): 269–278.

53. L. Fu et al., "Three new triterpenes from Nerium oleander and biological activity of the isolated compounds". *J. Nat. Prod., 68* (2) (2005): 198–206.

54. J. C. Steele et al., "*In vitro* and *in vivo* evaluation of betulinic acid as an antimalarial". *Phytother. Res., 13* (2) (1999): 115–119.

55. Z. Zhang et al., "Natural products inhibiting Candida albicans secreted aspartic proteases from Tovomita krukovii". *Planta Medica, 68* (1) (2002): 49–54.

56. C. A. Dehelean et al., "Study of the betulin enriched birch bark extracts effects on human carcinoma cells and ear inflammation". *Cem. Cent. J., 6* (1) (2012): 137.

57. C. Chandramu et al., "Isolation, characterization and biological activity of betulinic acid and ursolic acid from Vitex negundo L". *Phytother. Res., 17* (2) (2003): 129–134; F. Stephane & G. Marion, "Ursolic, oleanolic and betulinic acids: Antibacterial spectra and selectivity indexes". *J. Ethnopharmacol., 120* (2) (2008): 272–276.

58. C. Stapley, *The Tree Dispensary: The Uses, History, and Herbalism of Native European Trees* (London: Aeon Books, 2021).

59. T. Efferth et al., "The antiviral activities of artemisinin and artesunate". *Clin. Infect. Dis., 47* (6) (2008): 804–811.

60. T. Efferth et al., "The anti-malarial artesunate is also active against cancer". *Int. J. Oncol., 18* (4) (2001): 767–773.

61. M. Wood, *The Book of Herbal Medicine: Using Plants as Medicine* (Berkeley, CA: North Atlantic Books, 2004), pp. 233–241.

62. P. Saar-Reismaa et al., "Extraction and fractionation of bioactives from Dipsacus fullonum L. leaves and evaluation of their anti-Borrelia activity". *Pharmaceut. (Basel), 15* (1) (2022): 87.

63. M. Grieve, *A Modern Herbal: The Medicinal, Culinary, Cosmetic, and Economic Properties, Cultivation, and Folklore of Herbs, Grasses, Fungi, Shrubs, and Trees with All Their Modern Scientific Uses, Revised Edition* (Dorchester: Dorset Press, 1992).

64. Buhner, *Healing Lyme*, pp. 219–220.

65. Ibid., p. 307.

66. E. Sapi et al., "*Borrelia* and *Chlamydia* can form mixed biofilms in infected human skin tissues". *Eur. J. Microbiol. Immunol. (Bp), 92* (20) (2019): 46–55.

67. S. H. Buhner, *Natural Treatments for Lyme Coinfections: Anaplasma, Babesia, and Ehrlichia* (Rochester, VT: Healing Arts Press, 2015), p. 95.

68. E. Sapi et al., "*Borrelia* and *Chlamydia* can form mixed biofilms in infected human skin tissues". *Eur. J. Microbiol. Immunol. (Bp), 92* (20) (2019): 46–55; N. M. Atre & D. D. Khedkar, "A review on herbal remedies for sexually transmitted infections (STIs) from Melghat Region of Maharashtra State, India". *European J. Med. Plants, 31* (14) (2020): 1–17.

69. S. H. Buhner, *Herbal Antivirals: Natural Remedies for Emerging and Resistant Viral Infections* (North Adams, MA: Storey Publishing, 2013), pp. 192–208.

Chapter 6

1. L. Johnson et al., "Severity of chronic Lyme disease compared to other chronic conditions: A quality of life survey". *Peer J., 2* (2014): e322.

2. https://www.cdc.gov/parasites/babesiosis/gen_info/faqs.html

3. W. Rawls, *Unlocking Lyme: Myths, Truths, and Practical Solutions for Chronic Lyme Disease* (Cary, NC: FirstDoNoHarm Publishing, 2017), p. 347.
4. https://www.cdc.gov/bartonella/faq.html; https://www.cdc.gov/bartonella/index.html
5. S. H. Buhner, *Healing Lyme Disease Coinfections: Complementary and Holistic Treatments for Bartonella and Mycoplasma* (Rochester, VT: Healing Arts Press, 2013), pp. 345–347.
6. H. Khater, M. Govindarajan, & G. Benelli (Eds.), *Natural Remedies in the Fight Against Parasites* (Rijeka, Croatia: InTech, 2017).
7. M. D. Wells et al., "The medical leech: An old treatment revisited". *Microsurgery, 14* (3) (1993): 183–186.
8. Buhner, *Healing Lyme Disease Coinfections*, p. 307.
9. E. K. Benedikz et al., "Bacterial flagellin promotes viral entry via an NF-κB and Toll Like Receptor 5 dependent pathway". *Sci. Rep., 9* (2019): 7903; I. A. Hajam et al., "Bacterial flagellin – a potent immunomodulatory agent". *Exp. Mol. Med., 49* (9) (2017): e373.

Chapter 7

1. R. C. M. van Kruijsdijk et al., "Individualised prediction of alternate-day aspirin treatment effects on the combined risk of cancer, cardiovascular disease and gastrointestinal bleeding in healthy women". *Heart, 101* (5) (2015): 369–375.
2. A. Rosenblum et al., "Opioids and the treatment of chronic pain: controversies, current status, and future directions". *Exp. Clin. Psychopharmacol., 16* (5) (2008): 405–416.
3. K. Seibert et al., "Pharmacological and biochemical demonstration of the role of cyclooxygenase 2 in inflammation and pain". *Proc. Nat. Acad. Sci., 91* (25) (1994): 12013–12017.
4. S. Porges & S. Carter, *Polyvagal Theory, Oxytocin, and the Neurobiology of Love. Using the Body's Social Engagement System to Promote Feelings of Safety, Connectedness, Intimacy, and Recovery from Threat and Chronic Stress* (Professional Counselling & Psychotherapy Seminars, Ballintemple, Cork, Ireland, 2019).
5. C. R. Marinac et al., "Frequency and circadian timing of eating may influence biomarkers of inflammation and insulin resistance associated with breast cancer risk". *PLoS One, 10* (8) (2015): e0136240.
6. P. Hunter, "The inflammation theory of disease: The growing realization that chronic inflammation is crucial in many diseases opens new avenues for treatment". *EMBO Rep., 13* (11) (2012): 968–970.
7. J. M. Mullington et al., "Sleep loss and inflammation". *Best Pract. Res. Clin. Endocrinol. Metab., 24* (5) (2010): 775–784.
8. C. P. N. Watson et al., "The post-mastectomy pain syndrome and the effect of topical capsaicin". *Pain, 38* (1989): 177–186.
9. K. Mallion, *The CBD Handbook: Using and Understanding CBD and Medical Cannabis* (Lewes: Aeon Books, 2021).
10. J. Feng et al., "Selective essential oils from spice or culinary herbs have high activity against stationary phase and biofilm *Borrelia burgdorferi*". *Front. Med. (Lausanne), 4* (2017): 169.
11. Ibid.

12. Kate Parker is a medical herbalist (https://www.horsechestnutherbals.co.uk).
13. X. Ma et al., "Essential oils with high activity against stationary phase *Bartonella henselae*". *Antibiotics (Basel), 8* (4) (2019): 246.
14. *You Cannot Heal Trauma by Talking about Trauma* (https://www.instagram.com/p/BqnuA55A04S/); *The Freeze Trauma Response* (https://www.instagram.com/p/CTxcHeoPw_y/?hl=en-gb). See also N. LePera, *How to Do the Work: Recognize Your Patterns, Heal from Your Past, Create Your Self* (London: Orion Spring, 2021).
15. S. Porges, *The Polyvagal Theory: Neurophysiological Foundations of Emotions, Attachment, Communication, Self-Regulation* (New York: Norton, 2011).
16. A. Tynan et al., "Control of inflammation using non-invasive neuromodulation: past, present and promise". *Int. Immunol., 34* (2) (2022): 119–128; Y. Gidron et al., "The vagus nerve can predict and possibly modulate non-communicable chronic diseases: Introducing a neuroimmunological paradigm to public health." *J. Clin. Med., 7* (10) (2018): 371.
17. https://www.heartmath.co.uk

Chapter 8

1. T. Chevalley et al., "Arginine increases insulin-like growth factor-I production and collagen synthesis in osteoblast-like cells". *Bone., 23* (2) (1998): 103–109; P. Torricelli et al., "Human osteopenic bone-derived osteoblasts: Essential amino acids treatment effects". *Artif. Cells Blood Substit. Immobil. Biotechnol., 31* (1) (2003): 35–46.
2. T. Y. C. Tan et al.. "The health effects of chocolate and cocoa: A systematic review". *Nutrients., 13* (9) (2021): 2909.

Chapter 9

1. B. J. Diamond & M. R. Bailey, "Ginkgo biloba: Indications, mechanisms, and safety". *Psychiat. Clin. North. Amer, 36* (1) (2013): 73–83.

Chapter 10

1. C. A. Nelson et al., "Incidence of clinician-diagnosed Lyme disease, United States, 2005–2010". *Emerg. Infect. Dis., 21* (9) (2015): 1625–1631.
2. K. J. Kugeler et al., "Geographic distribution and expansion of human Lyme disease, United States". *Emerg. Infect. Dis., 21* (8) (2015): 1455–1457.
3. M. Citera et al., "Empirical validation of the Horowitz Multiple Systemic Infectious Disease Syndrome Questionnaire for suspected Lyme disease". *Int. J. Gen. Med., 10* (2017): 249–273 (Questionnaire: https://doyouhavelyme.com/online-test-form); R. Horowitz, *Why Can't I Get Better? Solving the Mystery of Lyme and Chronic Disease* (New York: St Martin's Press, 2013) (Questionnaire: https://cangetbetter.com/symptoms).
4. R. Dillon et al., "Lyme disease in the U.K.: Clinical and laboratory features and response to treatment". *Clin. Med. (London) 10,* (5) (October 2010): 454–457.
5. M. Dehhaghi et al., "Human tick-borne diseases in Australia". *Front. Cell. Infect. Microbiol., 9* (3) (2019): 1–17.

Lyme disease symptoms questionnaire

https://cangetbetter.com/wp-content/uploads/2020/11/BLP_MISIDSLymeQuestionnaire.pdf

Testing laboratories

ArminLabs GmbH   www.arminlabs.com
Zirbelstr. 58, 2. Stock, 86154 Augsburg, Germany
Email: info@arminlabs.com   Telephone: +49-821780-93150

Armin tests can be arranged through the Academy of Nutritional Medicine
   (https://aonm.org/armin-labs/)
Email: info@aonm.org   Telephone 0333-121-0305

Nordic labs
Nordic Laboratories, Nygade 6, 3 sal, 1164 Copenhagen K, Denmark
Email: info@nordic-labs.com   Telephone +45-33-75-10 00

The Doctor's Laboratory   www.tdlpathology.com/tests
76 Wimpole Street, London, W1G 9RT
Telephone 02073-077383

Support groups

Lyme Disease U.K.   https://lymediseaseuk.com

Royal College of General Practitioners   https://elearning.rcgp.org.uk/
Lyme disease toolkit: https://elearning.rcgp.org.uk/mod/book/view.php?id=12535

Lyme Disease Action   https://www.lymediseaseaction.org.uk

International Lyme and Associated Diseases Society   https://www.ilads.org

Lymedisease.org   https://www.lymedisease.org

Caudwell LymeCo Charity   http://caudwelllyme.com/contact

Polyvagal theory

Resources and articles   https://www.stephenporges.com

Herb suppliers

Neal's Yard Remedies   https://www.nealsyardremedies.com
2A Kensington Gardens, Brighton BN1 4AL
Telephone: 01273-601464

Integrative health   https://www.intergrativehealth.bio

Napier's   https://napiers.net

Pure Health Mushrooms   https://www.purehealthonline.co.uk/

Western Botanical Medicine   https://www.westernbotanicalmedicine.com
PO Box 1, Whitethorn, CA 95589, USA
Email: andrew@westernbotanicalmedicine.com   Telephone: +1-707-986-9506

Woodland Essence   www.woodlandessence.com
392 Teacup Street, Cold Brook, NY 13324, USA
Telephone +1-315-845-1515

Books

Healing Lyme: Natural Healing of Lyme Borreliosis and the Coinfections Chlamydia and Spotted Fever Rickett-siosis, 2nd Edition, by S. H. Buhner (Randolph, VT: Raven Press, 2015)

Healing Lyme Disease Coinfections: Complementary and Holistic Treatments for Bartonella and Mycoplasma, by S. H. Buhner (Rochester, VT: Healing Arts Press, 2013)

Herbal Antibiotics: Natural Alternatives for Treating Drug-Resistant Bacteria, 2nd Edition, by S. H. Buhner (North Adams, MA: Story Publishing, 2012)

Herbal Antivirals: Natural Remedies For Emerging & Resistant Viral Infections, 2nd Edition, by S. H. Buhner (North Adams, MA: Story Publishing, 2021)

Insights Into Lyme Disease Treatment: 13 Lyme-literate Health Care Practitioners Share Their Healing Strategies, by Connie Strasheim (South Lake Tahoe, CA: BioMed Publishing, 2009)

Natural Treatments for Lyme Coinfections: Anaplasma, Babesia, and Ehrlichiavz, by S. H. Buhner (Rochester, VT: Healing Arts Press, 2015)

Why Can't I Get Better? Solving the Mystery of Lyme and Chronic Disease Hardcover, by Richard I. Horowitz (New York: St. Martin's Press, 2013)

Further reading on Mushrooms

The Fungal Pharmacy: The Complete Guide to Medicinal Mushrooms & Lichens of North America, by Robert Rogers (Berkeley, CA: North Atlantic Books, 2011)

Medicinal Mushrooms: A Clinical Guide, by Martin Powell (Eastourne: Mycology Press, 2010)

Turkey Tail Mushrooms Help Immune System Fight Cancer, by Paul Stamets, 2012 (https://www.huffpost.com/entry/mushrooms-cancer_b_1560691)

INDEX

abdominal pain, 104, 140, 175
acesulfame, 195
acetylcholine (ACH), 85, 103, 190–192
acetylcholinesterase, 190
ACH (acetylcholine), 85, 103, 190–192
aches and pains, 56, 140, 180
acidophilus, 38
acid reflux, 148
acne, 75–76, 120
activated charcoal, 50
acupuncture, 45, 176
adaptogens, 55, 67, 114, 123, 132, 142, 159
addictive personalities, 170
adrenal dysfunction, 32
adrenaline, 190
    rush, 142, 160
agave, 218
air hunger, 32, 140, 142
ALA (alpha-linolenic acid), 196, 198, 208, 214
alkaloids, 80, 133, 158
allergic reactions, 83
allergic rhinitis, 99
allergies, 25, 31, 83, 92, 101, 120, 160, 173
Allium sativum (garlic), 50–52, 91–92, 148, 152, 155, 159,
        189, 226
Allium ursinum (wild garlic), 91
alpha-linolenic acid (ALA), 196, 198, 208, 214
alpha-lipoic acid, 148, 161
Alzheimer's disease, 89, 96, 103, 190
amarinth, 195
amino acid(s), 143, 154, 206, 215–216, 218, 220
amiodarone, 147
Ammi visnaga (khella), 147
amoebiasis, 93
amoxicillin, 28, 34, 38–40
amphetamine, 133
ampicillin, 76, 112
A-Myco-specific formulas, 150
anaemia, 68, 132–133, 212
    haemolytic, 141
anaesthesia, 106

analgesics, 65, 68, 80, 101, 108, 132, 159, 174, 176, 233
Anaplasma, 23
andrographis (*Andrographis paniculata*, Chuan Xin
        Lian, King of Bitters), 29, 52, 65–66, 152–153,
        158–159, 161, 191
angina, 70, 97, 147
    chest pain, 116
ankles, swollen, 31
anorexia, 140
antacids, 38
anthocyanins, 142, 199, 213, 215
anti-allergenics, 99
anti-Alzheimer's, 112
anti-anaemics, 67
anti-anxiety medication, 83
anti-arrhythmics, 85, 108, 127
anti-arthritics, 110, 125, 129
anti-atherosclerotics, 116
anti-Babesia activity, 117
antibacterial(s), 53, 55–56, 65, 70, 73, 78, 80, 83, 85, 89,
        91, 95, 99–101, 108, 110, 114, 116, 123, 125,
        127, 132, 135, 143, 146–147, 153, 159–161, 180,
        193, 225
antibiotic(s) [*passim*]:
    bactericidal, 40–41
    bacteriostatic, 40
    broad-spectrum, 41
    information on taking, 38–40
    intravenous, 39
        long-term, 37
    macrolide, 141
    natural, 37, 53–59
    overuse of, 53
    side effects, 48
antibiotic-resistant bacteria, 53
antibody tests(s)/testing (serology), 16, 21–23, 25
anticancer medications, 67–68, 70, 73, 83, 99, 101, 128
anticarcinogenics, 125, 159
anti-clotting agent, 92
anticoagulants, 9, 72, 80, 84, 92, 95, 116, 124, 180
anticonvulsants, 80, 83